Hi Valerie:

I am excited to share that my book is now published. I am delighted to send you a copy as an appreciation of your support and friendship.

I believe you will find it informative and enjoyable.

*[signature]*

# CURLY HAIR

## Structure, Properties, and Care

Ali Naqi Syed, PhD

Hasnia Publishing

# Curly Hair: Structure, Properties, and Care

### Ali Naqi Syed, PhD

| | |
|---|---|
| Cover Design: | Huma Akhtar |
| Illustrations: | Huma Akhtar |
| Primary Editor: | Maliha Syed |
| Secondary Editor: | Elisabeth J Kallos |
| Layout: | Maliha Syed |

Library of Congress Control Number: 2023914474
ISBN: 978-0-578-86659-8
1st Edition
Copyright © 2023 Hasnia Publishing

All rights reserved. Reproduction, distribution, or transmission of this book or any portion thereof in any form or by any means, including photocopying, microfilming, recording, or other electronic or mechanical methods, is strictly prohibited without prior written permission from the publisher, except in the case of brief quotations embodied in critical reviews and certain other noncommercial uses permitted by copyright law.

### NOTICE

The content of this book is based upon the research and the personal and professional experiences of the author. It is intended for informational purposes only and is not intended to diagnose, treat, cure, or prevent any condition or disease. The content of this book is not intended as a substitute for consulting with a healthcare professional. While the author has made best efforts to ensure the accuracy of the information contained in this book, the author and publisher will not be held responsible for any inaccuracies or omissions and expressly disclaim any and all liability, loss, or risk, whether personal or otherwise, arising directly or indirectly from the use or application of any information presented in this book. The mention of trade names or commercial products does not imply endorsement or recommendation by the author or publisher.

## Hasnia Publishing
## Oak Brook, IL, 60523

# Table of Contents

**Dedication,** vi

**Acknowledgements,** vii

**Chapter 1 - Introduction,** 1

**Chapter 2 - The Structure of Curly Hair,** 7

    Architecture, Structure, & Properties of the Cuticles, 8

    The Cuticle Sub-Layers, 12

    The Hair Fiber Cortex, 15

    Medulla, 26

    Definition of Terms, 27

    Summary, 32

    References, 34

**Chapter 3 - Hair Textures & Their Properties,** 37

    Type 1 (Straight) Textures, 38

    Type 2 (Wavy) Textures, 39

    Type 3 (Curly) Textures, 40

    Type 4 (Coily) Textures, 40

    Qualitative & Directional Relationship of Hair Type & Properties, 41

    Combing Type 3 & Type 4 Hair, 42

    Hair Elasticity Comparison of Type 1 & Type 4 Hair, 45

    Shape of Wavy & Curly/Coily Hair, 46

    Relationship of Cortical Cells & the Shape of Hair, 48

    The Number of Cuticle Layers in Various Hair Types, 49

Porosity of Types 1, 2, 3, & 4 Hair,   50

   Comparing the Hair Growth of Caucasian & African-Descent...

        ...Individuals,   53

   Static Charge on African-American Hair,   55

   Hair Shine,   56

   Moisture Content of Type 1 & Type 4 Hair,   56

   References,   58

**Chapter 4 - Scalp & Hair Growth: Hair Loss & Remedies,   61**

   The Scalp,   61

   Hair Follicle,   62

   The Shape of Hair,   65

   Hair Growth,   66

   Causes of Hair Loss,   71

   Treating Hair Loss and Hair Loss Remedies,   80

   Definition of Terms,   93

   References,   102

**Chapter 5 - Cleansing the Hair and Scalp,   107**

   The Purpose of Cleansing Products & Shampoos,   109

   Hair & Scalp Cleansing Practices of Caucasians...

        ...& African-Americans,   110

   Differences in Hair & Scalp by Hair Type & Ethnicity,   110

   Impact of Detergents on Hair & Scalp Integrity,   111

   Mitigating Deletrious Effects of Sodium Lauryl...

        ...Sulfate on the Skin,   114

   Evolution of Detergents in Cleansing Prodcuts, Types of...

        ...Detergents, & Their Impact on Hair & Scalp,   115

   Classification of Detergents,   116

   Hair & Scalp Prior to Shampooing,   130

   The Physics of Hair & Scalp Cleansing,   131

   The Effect of Detergents on the Hair,   132

   The Effect of Detergents on the Skin,   134

Mitigating Shampoo Damage, 135
The Product Development Process, 137
Types of Shampoos, 141
Conclusions, 152
Exhibit A, 154
References, 157

## Chapter 6 - Conditioning & Damage Remedies, 161

Causes of Hair and Scalp Damage, 162
Remedies for Hair Damage, 168
State of Hair & Scalp Before Conditioner Treatment, 177
Factors Influencing Penetration of Conditioners, 178
Types of Conditioners, 182
Scalp Care While Formulating Conditioners, 190
Conclusions, 190
References, 192

## Chapter 7 - Hair Styling & Maintenance, 195

Types of Styling Products, 195
Maintenance Products, 200
Styling Products for Chemically Straightened Hair, 205
References, 207

## Chapter 8 - Modifying Textured Hair Permanently, 209

Chemical Relaxing, 210
Deswelling of the Hair During the Relaxer Process, 218
Smoothing Treatments for Straightening Hair, 219
Permanent Waving, 221
Hair Coloring, 224
Hair Lightening/Bleaching, 228
Permanent Hair Coloring, 235
References, 243

**Index, 245**

**Notes, 255**

# Dedication

This book is lovingly dedicated to my late parents, Hasnia K. Syed and Ali Ather Syed, who worked hard to send me to college. They encouraged me to complete my education and saw with pride that I flourished in my profession. I wish you were here today to celebrate the completion of this book!

I want to thank my wife, Dure, for allowing me to take time away from the family to write this book. I also want to thank my daughter, Dr. Maliha Syed, for providing valuable comments and my sons, Hasan Syed and Jafar Syed, for all the love, encouragement, and support they provided during the writing of this book.

# Acknowledgements

Writing this book was an extraordinary exercise in sharing the knowledge that I have acquired regarding the African-descent hair and scalp. During this journey of learning the science of the hair and scalp, and in particular the science of the African-descent hair and scalp, many people have contributed to my knowledge over the years. I must acknowledge the African-American, African-European, and Brazilian hairstylists who persuaded me to think more about all textures of hair around the world. During my lectures to hairstylists in general, the questions posed were always instrumental in refining my understanding about textured hair. I also want to acknowledge independent African-American distributors in the United States for their support, collaboration, and furtherance of my career, not just as a chemist but also as an entrepreneur.

# CHAPTER 1

# Introduction

Few books have been written to date focusing on curly hair and hair types. Most of the books that do exist on this topic have been written either by consumers or professional hairstylists. In this book, I present the perspective of a hair chemist who has spent most of his life researching the structure, physics, and chemistry of curly hair; formulating new products to care for curly hair; and manufacturing these new products. Herein, the term curly hair will encompass wavy, curly, and coily hair types. Curly hair is unique in terms of its geometric shape and has unique properties when compared to its counterpart, straight hair. Therefore, combing, cleansing, conditioning, and styling curly hair requires detailed knowledge and special techniques that are quite different from those required for the care of straight hair.

In order to have a discussion about curly hair we have to understand how hair is categorized. Historically hair has been categorized by race, mainly Caucasian (straight to wavy), Asian (straight), and African (curly to coily). Given human migratory patterns over the past few centuries the ethnicity model is outdated and we are moving towards classifying hair more objectively. For example, recently, hair typing systems such as Andre Walker's have emerged that classify hair into four categories: Type 1 as straight hair, Type 2 as wavy hair, Type 3 as curly hair, and Type 4 as coily hair (see Chapter 3 for more details on Andre Walker's hair typing system). Throughout this text we will refer to hair interchangeably using the terms outlined in **Table 1.1**.

Table 1.1 *Hair fiber shape descriptors*

| Hair Type | Shape Description | Ethnicity |
|---|---|---|
| Type 1 | Straight | Caucasian, Mongolian, Asian, Japanese |
| Type 2 | Wavy | Hispanic, Caucasian |
| Type 3 | Curly, S-shaped | African-American, African-descent, Brazilian |
| Type 4 | Curly-to-coily, Coily, Spiraled, Z-shaped | African-American, African-descent, Brazilian |

In this book, I discuss the logic of hair typing with respect to hair shape, as well as combing, cleansing, conditioning, styling, maintenance, and the role of the scalp in hair growth. As both consumers and hairstylists are deeply involved in the art of curly hair involving all of the above-mentioned areas, it is my hope that they will benefit from the inner secrets of a formulating hair chemist, and gain an expanded understanding of curly hair and how to care for it on a daily or weekly basis. Every day, new products for curly hair are introduced, and it is important for consumers to know the parameters of evaluating these products.

In Chapter 2, the structure of hair is discussed in simple terms. The structure of the cuticles, the cell membrane complex (CMC) and its various types, and cortical cell types such as para- and ortho- cells are discussed with respect to hair type. The structural differences between Types 1, 2, 3, and 4 hair are described based on cortical-cell differences and the number of cuticle layers. The inner structure of the cortex is methodically examined, based on macrofibrils, microfibrils/intermediate filaments, the matrix, protofibrils, protofilaments, and dimers. Lastly, the role of the medulla is explained. At the end of the chapter, the terms used in discussing the structure of hair are defined.

In Chapter 3, hair types and the various properties associated with them are discussed. For example, with the stepwise change from Type 1 (straight) to Type 4 (coily) hair, a dramatic increase occurs in waviness, porosity, ellipticity, frizziness, shrinkage, twists in the hair strand, and scalp dryness. Similarly, in going from Type 1 to Type 4 hair, a negative association can be observed, namely, a declining trend in scalp moisture, strength or elasticity, shine, smoothness, layers of cuticles, 18-MEA, and hair growth.

Chapter 4 deals with the scalp and hair growth, followed by hair loss and its remedies. A comparison of the scalp's moisture content and its transepidermal water loss properties (TEWL) is presented, and the differences between Caucasian and African-descent hair are pointed out. The parts of a hair follicle and differences in follicle shape between Caucasian and African-descent hair are explained. The hair growth cycle is discussed, and the anagen, catagen, telogen, and exogen phases are detailed, along with differences in the hair growth rate among Caucasian and African-descent populations. The causes of hair loss such as androgenetic alopecia, traction alopecia, chemically induced alopecia, dandruff-caused alopecia, menopause, and dietary deficiencies are discussed. Lastly, hair loss remedies based on medical science such as minoxidil, finasteride, and dutasteride are presented and their side effects are described. Alternative remedies such as saw palmetto extract and phytosterols are introduced, and natural ingredients such as biotin; copper; green tea; aloe vera gel; iron; zinc; niacin; fatty acids; selenium; Vitamins D, E, and A; folic acid; and amino acids are described. Dandruff remedies and surgical transplants are briefly touched upon. The definition of terms used in the chapter is provided to help readers.

In Chapter 5, the cleansing of the hair and scalp is discussed in great detail. Cleansing plays a crtically important role in ensuring a healthy head of hair. The purpose of cleansing the hair and scalp is explained with reference to the differences between Caucasian and African-descent consumers. A number of relevant aspects are examined in this context such as moisture content and TEWL; the impact of detergents on hair and scalp integrity, notably with respect to moisture content and TEWL; and mitigation of the deleterious effects of detergents such as sodium lauryl sulfate. **Various types of detergents are described, including anionic, cationic, amphoteric, and natural detergents. Explained are the physics of hair and scalp cleansing and the effects of detergents on the pH of the hair and scalp, the moisture content and TEWL of the hair and scalp, as well as the integrity of hair surface lipids and the cuticles. Mitigation of hair and scalp damage is then reviewed.** In addition, a six-step product development process is described for hair chemists, hairstylists, consumers, and new entrepreneurs, highlighting the extensive efforts involved in the development of new products. Types of shampoos and co-wash cleansers are also discussed in detail.

In Chapter 6 the various ways to condition the hair and scalp and remedies for treating a damaged hair and scalp are outlined. First, the causes of hair damage are explored ranging from chlorine damage in swimmers' hair to damage from chemical treatments such as lightening, relaxing, and coloring. To mitigate damage, remedies must be based upon the proper selection of quaternary conditioning agents, according to the hair type and its needs, such as cationic silicone polymers, polyquaternium compounds, additives such as moisturizing agents, hair strengthening agents, hair pH balancers, and scalp rebuilders. The factors involved in the penetration of these conditioners into the hair and scalp such as length of application time, heat, and pH, along with the types of conditioners used are discussed in detail so that consumers can apply them in their everyday hair and scalp care practices in order to alleviate potential damages.

Chapter 7 provides a discussion of hairstyling and maintenance products, which are essential to the final appearance and assembly of curly hair. Styling products are based on leave-in conditioners and special waters containing essential oils, ceramides, and vitamins for the hair and scalp. These special waters are a new innovation in the field. Other hair styling products are twist and defining creams, curling jellies, curling creams, curling smoothies, and foam setting-lotions. Daily maintenance products for style preservation are moisturizing hair lotions, butter creams, natural oils (especially those rich in phytosterols), edge defining pomades, oil sheen sprays, and scalp serums. Scalp serums are particulary important for stimulating the scalp and discouraging the presence of fungi and bacteria on the scalp, which aids proper hair growth.

Last, but not least, Chapter 8 familiarizes the reader with products that modify the hair temporarily such as thermal straightening and systems that change the hair permanently such as hair relaxers, smoothing treatments, permanent waves, permanent hair colors, and hair lightening. Each permanent system for hair is discussed with its advantages and disadvantages, so that consumers can make informed decisions, based on scientific facts rather than marketing and advertising gimmicks.

Finally, this book has been a sincere effort of mine. It represents the culmination of my own journey of learning about curly hair and its associated scalp. The drawings of the structure of hair are our original renderings which were created from a comprehensive review of the current literature. The goal of this book is to offer the most current facts regarding the treatment of curly hair with appropriate products so the reader can make informed choices that will keep their hair and scalp beautiful and healthy forever.

# CHAPTER 2

# The Structure of Curly Hair

Daily grooming practices and the application of products for cleansing, conditioning, and styling the hair can cause changes in the hair structure. These changes can even amount to damage to the hair and scalp. In order to understand the causes of such damage, it is important to understand the structure of hair, which is very complex, and varies subtly between different hair types and ethnic groups. Thus, studying the structure of human hair becomes a very interesting science, and a plethora of literature is available regarding the structure of human hair. While many books and scientific articles have been published regarding the structure of hair, the effort of this book is based upon reviewing the literature and presenting it in a simple way so that the beginning hair chemist, hairstylist, and consumer can easily understand the structure of hair before they delve into the field of hair care.

As defined in various chemistry books and all of the relevant literature, hair is composed of a water-insoluble protein, known as keratin, and, by virtue of being a protein, keratin consists of many amino acids as its basic units. The physical shape of hair has mainly three parts: the cuticles, the cortex, and the medulla. A schematic of the structure of a human hair fiber is shown in **Figure 2.1**, where each component and its respective dimensions are specified. Each part of the hair is very complex in its own right and will be explained in detail in this chapter.

**Cuticles.** The cuticles form a protective layer around the outer surface of the hair fiber. According to Swift (1999, p. 24), there are six to ten layers of cuticles present on the surface of a hair fiber. According to Leon (1972), these cuticle layers are glued together with a cell membrane complex, simply referred to as CMC (p. 432). The cuticle layers differ in number in curly/coily hair; there are only two cuticle layers on the outer side of the crimp of curly/coily hair (p. 435).

**Cortex and medulla.** The inside of the hair consists of the cortex. In certain hair types, the very center of the hair contains a discontinuous empty space called the medulla. Fine and thin hair may not contain a medulla. The cortex is composed of spindle-shaped cortical cells (para- and ortho-), glued together with a cell membrane complex, adhesion proteins, and lipids. A cortical cell contains macrofibrils that are embedded in an intermacrofibrilar matrix, simply referred to as the matrix. Inside a macrofibril are microfibrils, also known as intermediate filaments (IFs), which possess the finest, most intricate cylindrical and helical structure. These IFs are in turn embedded in a macrofibril via a hydrophilic (i.e., water-loving), sulfur-rich protein matrix.

The schematic of the structure of hair, shown in **Figure 2.1**, illustrates to what magnitude the hair fiber diameter increases from one of the smallest parts of the hair (i.e., the dimer) to the other parts of the hair fiber in ranges that stretch from the nanometer scale to the micrometer scale. According to Leon (1972), a dimer is two nanometers in diameter (p. 433), whereas the human hair fiber as a whole is 75–80 micrometers on average. Thus, the diameter of the hair fiber as a whole is roughly 40,000 times larger than the diameter of a dimer.

## Architecture, Structure, & Properties of the Cuticles

Robbins (2002) explained that the outermost surface of a hair fiber is composed of cuticles and that five to ten layers of these cuticles

*Curly Hair: Structure, Properties, & Care* — **Chapter 2**

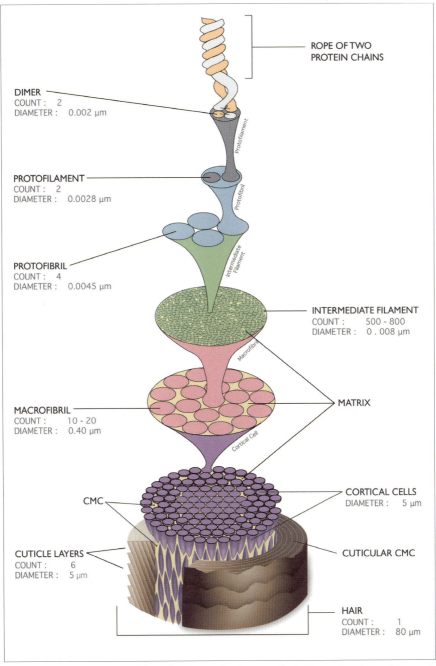

Figure 2.1. Schematic of the structure of a human hair fiber, showing all important components and their dimensions.

envelop the hair shaft in order to protect the hair from all sorts of potential damage (p. 25). The architecture of the cuticle layers of a hair fiber is shown in **Figure 2.2**. The cuticles are like shingles on a roof, and, like shingles, they overlap to form a thick protective mass of five to ten layers. The mass of these shingles offers resistance to penetration by undesirable environmental elements and large molecules. According to Swift (1999), there are approximately ten layers of cuticles at the root end, and then the number of cuticle layers decreases toward the tip end of the hair fiber. This decrease in the number of cuticle layers is attributed to mechanical attrition, or wear and tear, and to the weathering effects of sunlight, combing and brushing, shampooing, chemical treatments, and other hairstyling techniques utilized by hairstylists and individuals at home (p. 24).

According to Franbourg and Leroy (2005), each cuticle layer is

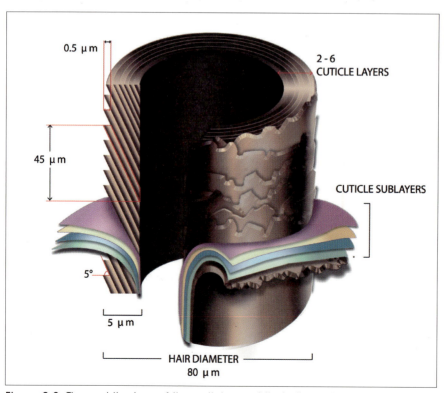

Figure 2.2. The architecture of the cuticles and their dimensions. Adapted from Alan J. Swift (1999) Journal of Cosmetic Science, 50, p. 24.

approximately 45 microns (μm) long and 0.5 μm thick (p. 4). Swift (1999) reported that the length of the overlap area of one cuticle layer over another is approximately 5.0 μm and that each cuticle layer is approximately 60 μm² with rounded corners (p. 23). The wool literature reports that cuticles are rectangular with a length of 30 μm, a width of 20 μm, and a thickness of 0.5 μm (Hocker, 2002, p. 67). The architecture of the cuticle layers in terms of geometric arrangement in human hair is shown in **Figure 2.2**. According to Leon (1972), African-descent curly hair has a varying number of cuticle layers along the hair shaft, where only one to two cuticle layers are found on the outer side of the crimp where the hair is curving, and six to ten layers on the inner side of the crimp of a curved hair fiber (p. 435). The major (outer side of crimp) and minor (inner side of crimp) axes of the cross-section of hair fiber are shown in Figures 2.9 and 2.10 under the subheading Fiber Ellipticity, in a later section. The cuticles are also rich in the amino acid cystine and in some fatty acids. Evans et al. (1985) first discovered the presence of the fatty acid 18-methyleicosanoic acid (18-MEA) on the outermost surface of the cuticle, also known as the F layer. According to Jones et al. (1996), all of the 18-MEA is present on the uppermost surface of the cuticle cell membrane, but not in the lower beta layer (p. 461). According to Breakspear et al. (2005), African-American hair has less 18-MEA on the uppermost surface of the cuticle than Caucasian hair (p. 241). From this research, it can be deduced that a cuticle surface that is covered with a lower amount of 18-MEA would allow water and water-soluble substances such as reactive chemicals to penetrate faster into the cortex.

**Cell membrane complex (CMC).** Each cuticle layer is glued to the next cuticle layer with the help of a material called the intercellular cement or the cell membrane complex (CMC) and its intercellular spaces.

**Types of CMC.** There are three types of CMC. The first type is just between the cuticles, the second type is between the innermost cuticle layer and the outermost cortical cells, and the third CMC is between the cortical cells themselves. These three CMCs are somewhat different in their composition, which is further explained by Robbins (2009, p. 437).

- *Cuticle-cuticle CMC.* The essential role of the CMC between the cuticles is to help cohere one cuticle layer to the next layer.

- *Cuticle-cortex CMC.* This type of CMC provides cohesion between the innermost cuticle layer and the outermost cortical cells of the cortex. This cuticle-cortex CMC is more easily damaged by treatment with solvents than the cuticle-cuticle CMC, but not as much as the cortex-cortex CMC (Robbins, 2009, p. 446).

- *Cortex-cortex CMC.* The third type of CMC keeps the cortical cells glued together. This cortex-cortex CMC is more easily damaged by solvents, as compared to the cuticle-cuticle CMC and the cuticle-cortex CMC (Robbins, 2009, p. 447). The three CMCs are somewhat different in their behavior toward solvents.

The spaces within the CMC are the preferred route of penetration into the hair cortex and diffusion by many substances (Franbourg & Leroy, 2005, p. 14). The structure of these spaces in the CMC is still unknown. Reactive chemicals like relaxers, permanent colors, hair lighteners, and permanent waves attack the lipids of the CMC. The degradation of the CMC between the cuticles may cause the cuticle layers to unravel, weaken faster, and not play an effective role as a cortex protectant.

## The Cuticle Sub-Layers

The structure of a cuticle layer, shown in **Figure 2.3**, is quite complex. Each cuticle layer is further divided into four sublayers: the epicuticles, the A layer, the exocuticles, and the endocuticles.

**Epicuticle.** The epicuticle is a very thin membrane that covers the cuticle as its outermost layer. It is approximately five to seven nanometers (nm) thick and visible only in a transmission electron microscope (Franbourg & Leroy, 2005, p. 5). It is very hydrophobic in nature.

The F layer, which is composed of the fatty acid 18–MEA, covers the hair surface and is not very resistant to relaxers, permanent coloring agents, and hair lighteners on prolonged exposure. Significant chemical

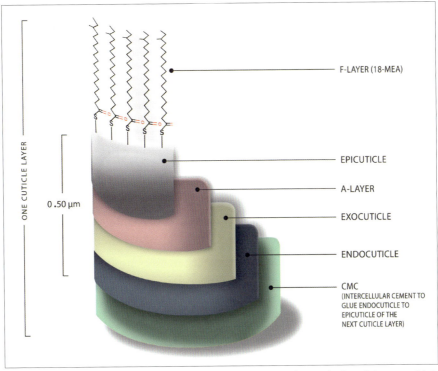

Figure 2.3. The sublayers of the cuticle layer. Also shown is the F layer, which is attached to the uppermost cuticle layer. The bottom layer of cuticle CMC is between the endocuticle and the epicuticle sublayer of the next cuticle.

changes take place in the epicuticle layer, thus rendering hair fibers more porous, and increasing interfiber friction. African-descent hair has less 18–MEA present on the fiber surface, compared to untreated Caucasian hair (Breakspear et al., 2005, p. 241).

**The A layer.** The A layer exists below the epicuticle layer. The A layer and exocuticle layer form approximately two thirds of the scale structure of the cuticles. They have a very high cystine content; the A layer contains approximately 35% cystine. Chemical analysis of the A layer also shows a high content of amino acids such as lysine and glutamic acid, suggesting the presence of isopeptide bonds, which further explains the A **layer's strong cro**ss-linkage structure (Jones et al., 2007, p. 341). The A layer resists attack by physical forces such as repetitive combing, blow-drying, and chemical forces such as alkalis, reducing agents, oxidizing agents, and proteolytic enzymes, which would be devastating to the integrity of the hair fiber without the cuticle's protection.

**Exocuticle.** The sublayer under the A layer is called the exocuticle; it has approximately 15% cystine content (Franbourg & Leroy, 2005, p. 5). The exocuticles do not have a fibrillar structure. The A layer is a part of the exocuticles, which are divided into the A layer and the B layer. The term B layer is usually what is meant by the term exocuticles.

**Endocuticle.** The endocuticle layer lies below the exocuticle layer and has a low content of cystine, approximately 3%. It is mechanically the weakest component of the cuticle structure. The gap in the cystine content between the endocuticles (3%) and the exocuticles (15%) is sizable. Due to the very low cystine content, the endocuticle layer has a very soft and deformable structure, and swells considerably more in water than the exocuticle layer. The cuticles become more pronounced in the wet state because of this water-induced swelling of the endocuticle layer. The entanglements between hair fibers are also greater in the wet state because of the extraordinary swelling of the endocuticles (Feughelman, 1997, p. 3). The endocuticle layer can easily deteriorate due to proteolytic agents and other reactive chemicals such as alkalis. The special advantage of the endocuticle layer may be that it offers some degree of protection by providing a cushion underneath the exocuticle layer from forces applied to the surface of the hair, such as combing, brushing, and blow-drying (Swift, 1999, p. 28).

Thus, the role of the cuticles is to oppose the penetration of reactive and nonreactive chemicals into the cortex of the hair and also to provide protection of the fiber during repeated combing and brushing (Wortman & Kure, 1994, p. 155). This protective role of the cuticles is a blessing for the long-term survival of the hair fiber. The cuticles also oppose the bending of the hair fiber to almost 74%, where 66% of this resistance is due to the exocuticles, and 8% is attributed to the endocuticles (Swift, 2000, p. 38). Therefore, to make fine hair thicker, the endocuticles should be stiffened via deposits of certain polymers, and coarse hair can be made softer by reducing the stiffness of the exocuticles.

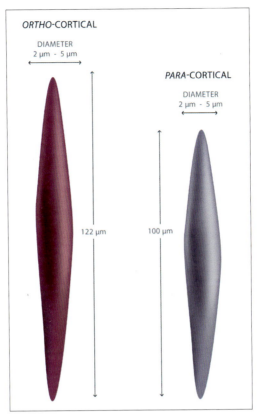

Figure 2.4. Shape and dimensions of a paracortical and an orthocortical cell.

## The Hair Fiber Cortex

The central core of the hair is called the cortex. It occupies 75% to 80% of the hair's volume and is covered by the cuticle layers. It is the mechanical powerhouse of the hair and is largely responsible for the hair fiber's elasticity and tensile strength (Feughelman, 1997, p. 3).

**Cortical cells.** The cortex is primarily composed of cortical cells, which are proteinaceous cells of elongated shape of regular and irregular cross-sections. The shape and dimensions of the cortical cells are shown in **Figure 2.4**.

The diameter of these cells is approximately 5 μm (Leon, 1972, p. 433), where paracortical cells are 100 μm in length but may decrease in length in wavy and curly/coily hair. Orthocortical cells are longer than paracortical cells. Higher curvature in hair is significantly related to the shorter length of the paracortical cells (Harland, et al. 2018, p. 5).

**Cortex-cortex CMC.** Each cortical cell is separate from its neighbor and the cells are glued together with the cortex-cortex CMC, which is ~25 nm thick (Feughelman, 1997, p. 3). The CMC of the cortex is made up of modified membranes of the original living cells, with intercellular adhesion provided by a laid-down intercellular cement, i.e., the cortex-cortex CMC.

Cuticle and cortical cells are glued together with the cuticle-cortex CMC. The cortical cells are glued to one another with the cortex-cortex CMC to form a composite, as shown in **Figure 2.5**.

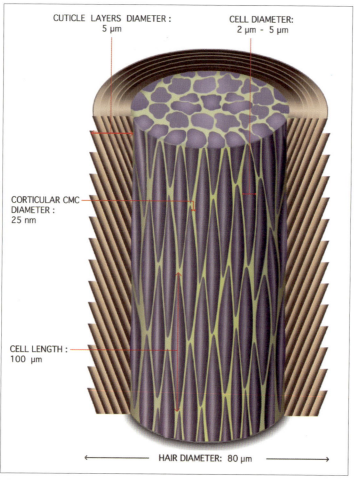

Figure 2.5. Positioning and dimensions of cortical cells within a hair fiber.

## Curly Hair: Structure, Properties, & Care    Chapter 2

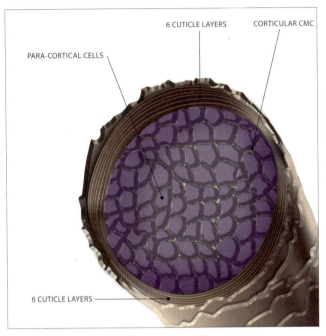

Figure 2.6. Type 1 straight hair has only paracortical cells.

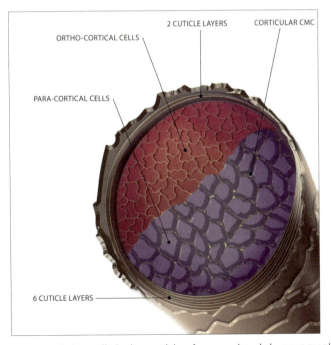

Figure 2.7. Type 4 curly-to-coily hair consists of approximately an equal number of rows of paracortical and orthocortical cells.

The cortex of a hair fiber appears uniform under an optical microscope, and no indication of boundaries of the cortical cells is discernible. To see the full details of the cortical cell structure, a scanning electron microscope must be used (Feughelman, 1997, p. 4).

Straight, Type 1 (Caucasian/Oriental/Mongolian-East Asian) hair tends to be composed of all paracortical cells, which are more uniform in diameter and shape, as shown in **Figure 2.6**.

According to Hocker (2002), paracortical cells contain cytoplasmic residues and nuclear remnants (p. 72). They have more cystine (~5%) and are more heat stable. Consequently, the hair is straight in shape and relatively uniform in diameter with an ellipticity of 1.22. African-descent hair, which is curly to coily in shape, consists of half paracortical cells and half orthocortical cells (~3% cystine); the latter are inherently irregular in shape and size. Cytoplasmatic residues and nuclear remnants are rarely present in orthocortical cells. Because African-descent hair has an equal number of rows of para- and orthocortical cells (**Figure 2.7**), it is curly in

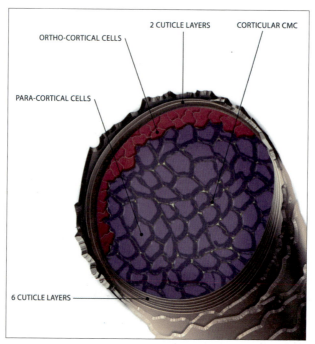

Figure 2.8. Type 2, Type 3A, Type 3B, wavy hair consists of mostly paracortical cells and a narrow row of orthocortical cells.

shape and displays a high degree of diameter variation along the hair shaft. Thus, African-descent hair displays very high ellipticity, ranging from 1.0 to 3.25 (Syed et al., 2013, p. 259). The African-descent hair follicle is concave in shape at the bulb and consists of different genes than straight hair, thus producing a curly to coily hair fiber (Westgate et al., 2017, p. 485).

Shown in **Figure 2.8**, mixed-race, curly hair (Type 2 and Types 3A & B) tends to have predominantly paracortical cells with a narrow row of orthocortical cells. Mixed-race hair is considered wavy to moderately curly

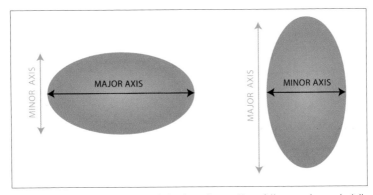

Figure 2.9. Fiber ellipticity is calculated as the ratio of the major axis (diameter) of a hair fiber to the minor axis (diameter).

and is more uniform in diameter along the hair shaft, compared to coily Type 4 hair. Type 2 and Type 3 hair is very difficult to straighten with alkali metal hydroxides, compared to Type 4 hair. This may be due to the predominance of paracortical cells with a higher cystine content (5%) than orthocortical cells (3%). On the paracortical side of the hair, the overall thickness of the cuticles is higher than on the orthocortical side (Kassenbaum, 1981, p. 60).

**Fiber ellipticity.** Hair fibers are not perfectly cylindrical in shape. Instead, they take on an oval or egg-shaped form. Ellipticity describes the three-dimensional shape of the hair fiber and denotes the ratio of the fiber diameter along two axes, as shown in **Figure 2.9**. Hair fibers have a major axis, which is the larger diameter, and a minor axis, which is the smaller diameter. Fiber ellipticity is calculated as the ratio of the major axis to the minor axis. Thus, if a hair fiber is cylindrical in shape, fiber ellipticity ~ 1.

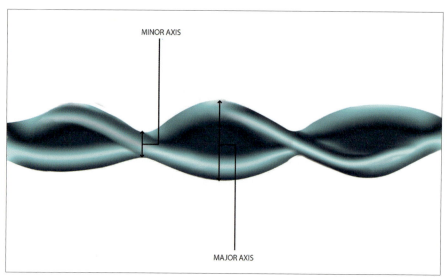

**Figure 2.10.** Twisted and coiled shape of curly-to-coily, African-descent hair fibers. The ellipticity of curly hair continues to change at various points along the hair shaft. The major axis shifts to becoming the minor axis and vice versa along the fiber shaft when fiber diameters (X and Y axis) are scanned throughout the fiber length.

However, the more ovoid the shape of the hair fiber, the higher the fiber ellipticity, >>1.

The ellipticity of human hair varies according to the extent of paracortical cells and orthocortical cells present. For example, the all-paracortical-cell hair of Type 1 displays ellipticity values of 1.22 to 1.44, whereas hair fibers with equal number of para- and orthocortical cells (i.e., African-descent hair fibers) displays higher ellipticity values of 1.895 and higher (Kamath et al., 1984, p. 25). Fibers that display high ellipticity are intricately twisted and coiled in shape and consist of many narrow spots along the hair shaft, as shown in **Figure 2.10**.

Curly-to-coily, African-descent hair fibers, in which the major and minor axes change frequently, form bottleneck-narrow stress points along the hair shaft. Thus making these fibers quite prone to breakage during grooming, where breakge is thought to occur at the narrow stress points along the fiber shaft. Fibers in which the minor axis is very narrow along the hair shaft break easily, even at low stress values. It is common knowledge that Type 4, African-descent hair breaks under much less stress than

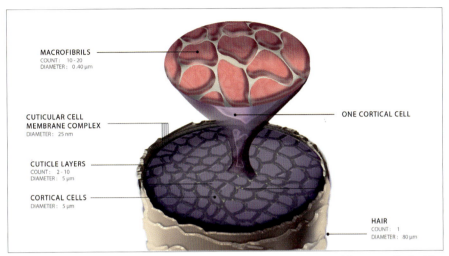

Figure 2.11. Each cortical cell contains approximately 10 to 20 macrofibrils. The diameter of a macrofibril is approximately 0.10–0.40 μm.

Type 1 (Caucasian or Asian) straight hair (Syed et al., 1995, p. 48).

**Macrofibrils.** Cortical cells consist of 10 to 20 macrofibrils, which are separated by a thin membrane within the cortical cell (Hocker, 2002, p. 72). These membranes also contain the pigment of the hair known as melanin, which is variably dispersed in the membrane. Macrofibrils are embedded in the cortical cells as units and are separated by intermacrofibrilar material or matrix in the cortical cells (Leon, 1972, p. 433). Rod-like structures, macrofibrils have a length of a few microns (μm) and a diameter of 0.1-0.4 μm (Franbourg & Leroy, 2005, p. 8). These keratinized macrofibril units are oriented longitudinally within the cells, thereby providing a very strong fiber-matrix composite, as shown in **Figure 2.11**.

**Microfibrils/Intermediate filaments (IFs).** Macrofibrils contains many microfibrils, also known as intermediate filaments (IFs). As seen through an electron microscope, a macrofibril consists of 500 to 800 long, uniform filaments called microfibrils. As shown in **Figure 2.12**, these microfibrils are oriented parallel to the axis of the hair fiber and are embedded in the macrofibrils. Microfibrils are approximately 8 nm or 0.008 μm in diameter (Parry & Steinert, 1999, p. 100). They are approximately 11 nm apart in wet fibers (Franbourg & Leroy, 2005, p. 44). Microfibrils

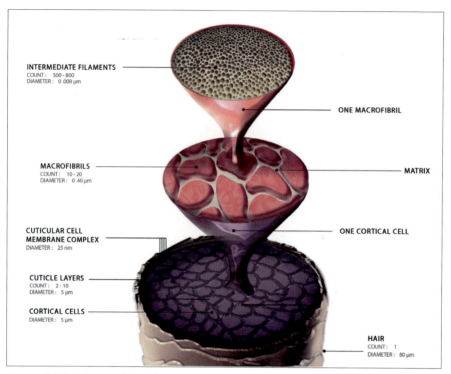

Figure 2.12. Intermediate filaments (IFs), or microfibrils, present in each macrofibril. Each IF is surrouded by the matrix shown above.

contain very organized helical material and are made of Type I and Type II keratins.

**The matrix.** Each microfibril (IF), is surrounded by an amorphous space called the matrix, show in in **Figure 2.12**. The matrix is composed of proteins high in sulfur content also known as keratin associated proteins (KAPs) (Shimomura & Ito, 2005, p. 230). The major role of the matrix is to keep the microfibrils in place and intact. More than 80 KAPs have been isolated from human hair and classified into more than 20 families. They represent ultrahigh sulfur KAPs, high sulfur KAPs, and high glycine/tyrosine KAPs (Rogers, et al. 2006, p. 215). If the matrix proteins (KAPs) are denatured, either partially or fully, the hair fiber seems to lose its mechanical strength (tensile strength and elasticity) proportionately. The loss in elasticity/tensile strength of hair fibers during chemical treatments seems to correspond to the extent of damage to the matrix proteins (KAPs).

# Curly Hair: Structure, Properties, & Care — Chapter 2

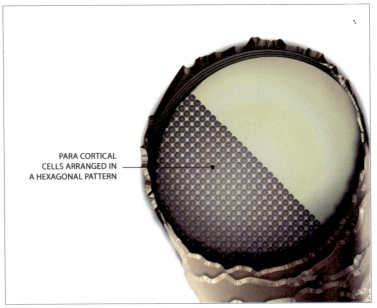

**Figure 2.13.** Cross-section of a Type 1 straight, Caucasian hair fiber showing the microfibrils in the paracortical cells arranged in a regular hexagonal pattern.

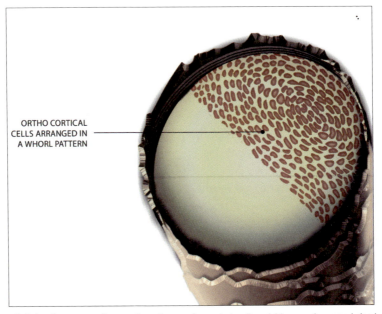

**Figure 2.14.** Cross-section of a Type 4 curly/coily, African-descent hair fiber showing the microfibrils within the orthocortical cells arranged in a whorl or spiral pattern.

Within paracortical cells, microfibrils are arranged in a regular hexagonal pattern, as shown in **Figure 2.13**. This hexagonal arrangement of the microfibrils in paracortical cells is responsible for the straightness of Type 1, Caucasian and Mongoloid hair fibers (Feughelmann, 1997, p. 6).

Orthocortical cells in African-descent hair are arranged in a whorl or spiral form, as shown in **Figure 2.14** (Nagase et al., 2008, p. 328). The orthocortical cells in the outer region of the crimp of curly hair are responsible for the curly configuration of the hair fiber, as in Type 3 and Type 4 curly/coily African-descent and Afro-Euro/Asian mixed-race hair. An example of the latter would be Brazilian hair with tremendous racial diversity. Japanese women with curly hair have both para- and orthocortical cells in certain proportions, making the hair wavy, as previously described.

Paracortical cells contain more cystine and are more heat stable than orthocortical cells. The introduction of significantly more orthocortical cells in Type 4 curly/coily (African-descent) hair makes it more vulnerable to chemical attack than its counterpart, Type 1 straight (Asian- and European-descent) hair. Even Type 2 wavy, mixed-race hair with predominantly paracortical cells and a narrow row of orthocortical cells is more resistant to chemical modifications such as hair straightening and other procedures. Normally, hair straighteners with higher concentrations of alkalis are effectively designed to straighten racially diverse hair, rather than Type 4 curly/coily (African-descent) hair.

**Protofibrils.** Microfibrils consist of four protofibrils. The structure of a protofibril is shown in **Figure 2.15**.

**Protofilaments.** There are two protofilaments in a protofibril. The structure of a protofilament is shown in **Figure 2.15**. Each protofilament consists of two dimers, also known as a tetramer. The diameter of a protofilament is 2.8 nm or 0.0028 µm (Hocker, 2002, p. 68). The protofilaments are the alpha-helical formations of two keratin proteins (Type I with acidic amino acid residues, and Type II with basic amino acid residues), which arrange themselves to form a helical rope. The association of eight protofilaments in four protofibrils forms the hexagonal structure of the microfibril/IF. There are approximately eight protofilaments in a microfibril; the remaining space in an IF consists of the intermicrofibril

*Curly Hair: Structure, Properties, & Care* **Chapter 2**

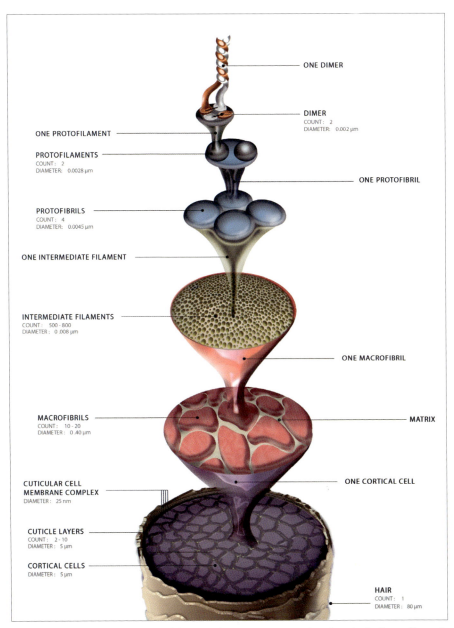

**Figure 2.15.** A schematic of the various components of a hair fiber. The dimensions of each component are also highlighted. In the top section, the four protofibrils in an IF are shown. Next, the two protofilaments in a protofibril are shown. The structure of a dimer is shown as the smallest component of the hair fiber, where two dimers make up one protofibril. The dimer is composed of two protein chains roped together.

matrix in which these protofilaments are embedded.

**Dimers.** A protofilament consists of two dimers; the structure of a dimer is shown in **Figure 2.15**. A dimer has two protein chains, roped together in a special helical pattern. There are four protofibrils, eight protofilaments (tetramers), and 16 dimers in a microfibril/IF. Therefore, there is a total of 32 protein chains of Type 1 and Type 2 proteins in an IF.

## Medulla

The discontinuous empty space that exists in the middle of a hair fiber is called the medulla. The shape of the medulla in human hair is shown in the scanning electron microscope (SEM) micrograph in **Figure 2.16**. While the function of the medulla is not well understood, and little research has been conducted to elucidate its chemistry and properties, the medulla is believed to contribute to greater volume and body in hair. The medulla may provide thermoregulatory properties to the hair with regard to the airspaces within the medulla. Hair fibers that are fine in texture seems to have very little or no medulla and tend to have very little body as well. Hair fibers that are coarse in texture seems to have a greater presence of medulla and, consequently, more body. Thus, the size of the medulla

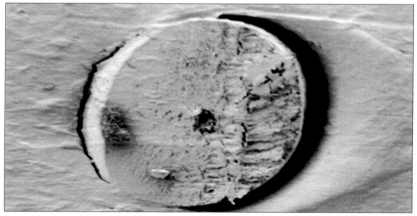

Figure 2.16. Scanning electron microscope (SEM) micrograph illustrating the shape of the medulla in the cross-section of a coarse hair fiber (x1550). The medulla can be seen in the very center of the cross-section as a hole or empty space in the hair fiber. Source: Courtesy of Avlon® Research Center.

determines the degree of body and volume of the hair.

## Definition of Terms

**A layer.** The second sublayer in a cuticle layer. It contains appoximately 35% cystine. Chemical analysis of the A layer shows the presence of large amounts of amino acids such as lysine and glutamic acid.

**Amino acids.** Organic compounds consisting of amino groups ($NH_2$) and acid groups (COOH). Twenty amino acids and a dimer of an amino acid appear to be all there is of these compounds in our universe.

**Angstrom (Å).** An internationally recognized unit, equivalent to a length of 0.1 nanometers or $1\times10^{-10}$ meters. It is sometimes used in expressing the size of an atom, the length of a chemical bond, and wavelength of visible-light spectra. It is commonly applied in structural biology. It is named after Anders Jonas Ångström.

**Cell membrane complex (CMC).** The glue keeping cuticles, cuticles and cortex, and cortical cells together. The essential role of CMC is to provide cohesion through adhesion proteins.

**Cortex.** The central core of the hair. It is covered by the cuticles and makes up ~75% to 80% of the hair volume. It is mechanically the most important part of the hair and largely responsible for the elasticity and tensile strength of the hair.

**Cortical cells.** The cortex is primarily made up of cortical cells, which are proteinaceous cells of elongated shape with regular or irregular cross-sections. The diameter of these cells is between 2 and 5 μm. The length of a cortical cell is approximately 100 μm (see **Figure 2.4**).

**Cross-section.** When hair is cut across and viewed from the top, the circumference of the cut depicts the cross-section of the hair.

**Cuticle layers.** The outermost surface of the hair is composed of cuticles; there are 6 to 10 layers of cuticles around the hair shaft to protect the hair from various kinds of damage. Curly hair may have only two layers on the outer side of the crimp.

**Elastic region.** The region on the stress/strain curve of a hair fiber where the hair fiber stretches in proportion to the force applied. The elastic region is up to 2% strain of the hair length, ideally.

**Elasticity.** Elasticity is the hair's response to the force required to extend the fiber by up to 2% of its length. The hair fiber extends linearly up to 2% of its length; this is called the elastic region, or Hookean region. After 2% extension, hair does not extend linearly anymore, but extends quite a bit with little force. When hair extends too much or unproportionally in response to a small force, the region is called yield region. After about 30% extension, the fiber again extends more steeply and, then, finally breaks. The force required to break the fiber is called break strength, or tensile strength, as shown in **Figure 2.17**, which depicts a typical stress-strain curve of a human hair fiber.

**Ellipticity.** The ratio of the major diameter to the minor diameter of a hair fiber (see **Figure 2.9**), indicating how cylindrical or ovoid the

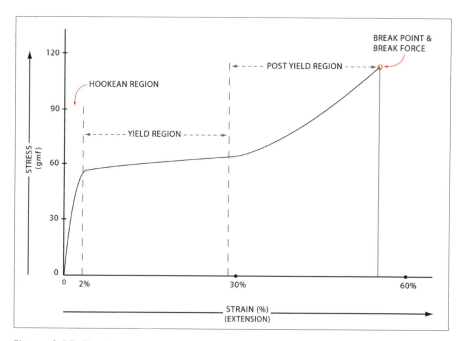

Figure 2.17. The stress-strain curve of a human hair fiber.

three-dimensional shape of the hair fiber.

**Endocuticle.** The endocuticle layer lies next to the exocuticle (B layer) and has a low cystine content of approximately 3%. It is mechanically the weakest component of the cuticle structure and swells like a sponge when wet.

**Epicuticle.** The epicuticle layer is a very thin membrane that covers the cuticle as the outermost layer. It is approximately 5-7 nm thick.

**Exocuticle.** The exocuticle layer is the sublayer below the A layer. It is called either the exocuticle or exocuticle B. It contains a cystine content of ~15% and does not have a fibrillar structure.

**External lipids of hair.** These external lipids are secreted by the sebaceous glands and gradually travel along the hair shaft, accounting for ~6% of the hair mass.

**Glycine.** An amino acid with the formula $NH_2CH_2COOH$. This amino acid is part of the matrix proteins in the hair fiber, also known as KAP.

**Heterodimers.** A dimer has two protein chains roped together in a special helical pattern as shown in **Figure 2.15**. There are 16 dimers in a microfibril/intermediate filament.

**Hydrogen bonding.** A hydrogen ion (+ve charge) of the amino group of one polypeptide forms an attractive interaction with a oxygen atom (-ve charge) of the carbonyl group of the opposing polypeptide. This weak bond is called a hydrogen bond, and the phenomenon is known as hydrogen bonding.

**Hydrophilic.** A substance that is water-loving and has a special affitinity for water.

**Hydrophilic sulfur-rich proteins.** The proteins of the matrix where microfibrils are embedded are very high in sulfur content. These proteins are hydrophilic in nature as well, and this is where much of the hair moisture resides. The high-sulfur proteins of the matrix are also called

KAP; they are high in glycine-tyrosine (HGT) proteins.

**Hydrophobic.** A substance that is water-repelling. These substances tend to be non-polar.

**Intermacrofibrilar matrix.** The matrix of the cortex where macrofibrils are embedded is known as the intermacrofibrillar matrix.

**Intermediate filament (IF).** Located inside a macrofibril, IFs are long, uniform filaments oriented parallel to the fiber axis. The old name for an intermediate filament was "microfibril". IFs are appoximately 8 nm, or 80 Å, or 0.008 μm, in diameter. They are spaced ~11 nm apart in wet fibers (see **Figure 2.12**). IFs contain very organized helical material consisting of Type 1 and Type 2 keratins.

**Internal lipids of hair.** These lipids are present in the cell membrane complex, the epicuticles, and free lipids inside the hair fiber structure. Internal lipids account for approximately 1% to 3% of the hair mass and consist of fatty acids and polar lipids, including ceramides.

**Keratin fiber.** The microfibrils/IFs of the cortex consist of alpha-helical protein chains that are roped together several times. These keratin protein ropes are embedded in the cortex matrix. This assembly is known as keratin fiber.

**Macrofibril.** Rod-like structures that are a few microns long, and 0.1–0.4 μm in diameter. These keratinized macrofibril units are oriented longitudinally within the cells, thereby providing a very strong fiber-matrix composite, as shown in **Figure 2.11**.

**Matrix.** The matrix is of two types: One kind of matrix is the space in which the macrofibrils are embedded; it is known as the intermacrofibrilar matrix. The second kind is the space where microfibrils/IFs are embedded; it is known as the intermicrofibrilar matrix. The hair shows a predominance of intermicrofibrilar matrix, which, usually, is simply called the matrix. The high-sulfur proteins of the matrix are referred to as KAP; these are proteins high in glycine-tyrosine (HGT) amino acids. The total cortex proteins consist of 60% KAPs.

**Medulla.** The medulla is the intermittent empty space that exists in the middle of the fiber. It is sometimes called modula of hair.

**Microfibril.** See intermediate filament (IF).

**Micron (µm).** One micron is equal to 1 millionth of a meter, and 1 meter is equivalent to 3.281 feet.

**Nanometer (nm).** One nanometer is equal to 1 billionth of a meter.

**Orthocortical cell.** A type of cortical cell that is of irregular shape and size and responsible for the curliness of hair. They normally exist on the outer side of the crimp in curly hair. IFs in orthocortical cells are arranged in a whorl pattern, which potentially causes curliness in a hair fiber.

**Paracortical cell.** A type of cortical cell that is spindle-shaped and more uniform in diameter and shape than an orthocortical cell (**Figure 2.4**). Paracortical cells contain cytoplasmic residues and nuclear remnants.

**Peptide.** When the nitrogen atom of the amino group of one amino acid joins with the carbon atom of the acid group of another amino acid, a peptide bond is created. A water molecule is also produced as a by-product when two amino acids chemically link via a peptide bond.

**Polypeptide.** When more than two amino acids join together forming peptide bonds, this chain of amino acids is called a polypeptide. Therefore, a polypeptide consists of many peptide bonds. A polypeptide can be very long and composed of many amino acids.

**Protein.** A protein consists of many amino acids that are linked together via peptide bonds to form polypeptide chains. The polypeptide chains further arrange themselves into secondary and tertiary structures forming large, two- and three-dimensional macromolecules, also known as proteins. Hair protein is known as keratin.

**Protofibril.** A protofibril exits inside a microfibril/intermediate filament. It is composed of eight protein chains. There are four protofibrils in a microfibril. These four protofibrils join together in the form of a rope to endow elastic properties to the keratin fiber (**Figure 2.15**).

**Protofilament.** A protofilament is composed of two dimers. The structure of a dimer is shown in **Figure 2.15**. A dimer has two protein chains roped together in a special helical pattern.

**Proteolytic materials.** Chemicals that can break down proteinaceous materials. Examples of proteolytic materials are enzymes, alkalis, and acids. They modify the protein chains for better or for worse.

**Relative humidity (RH).** The amount of water vapor that exist in the air. For example, at 95% RH, the air contains an excessive amount of water vapor, which makes the air quite humid. Conversely, at 20% RH, a very small amount of water vapor is present, and the air feels relatively dry.

**Tensile strength of hair.** The tensile strength of hair is equal to the force required to stretch the hair fiber to a desired extension (**Figure 2.17**). If the fiber is extended until it breaks, it has reached the tensile strength breakpoint. If the fiber is extended to 20% of its length, then one has a tensile strength at 20% extension.

**Trace elements in hair.** The hair fiber contains very small quantities of elements such as sodium, potassium, magnesium, calcium, strontium, zinc, iron, manganese, mercury, cadmium, lead, arsenic, selenium, silicone, and phosphorus, which are called trace elements. The total amount of these trace elements in hair is less than 1%.

**Tyrosine.** Tyrosine is an amino acid with the formula $NH_2CHCOOHCH_2C_6H_4OH$. This amino acid is part of the matrix proteins in the hair fiber, known as KAP.

## Summary

As indicated in the introduction to this chapter, the hair fiber's structure is very complex, and there are subtle variations in the structure of hair of different hair types and ethnic groups. Thus, this chapter is replete with professional terms, chemical formulas, measurements on the nanometer and micrometer scale, and many explanatory drawings. Yet, a human hair can also be described simply as having three main sections. First, there is the protective outer layer, made up of several cuticle layers. Much like the shingles on a roof, cuticles overlap each other to form a thick protective mass that is strengthened and held together by a gluelike substance, called the intercellular cement or cell membrane complex (CMC). This CMC is found in the other sections of the hair fiber as well, albeit with a somewhat different chemical composition, but with a similar task, namely, to cement together the various parts and layers of each section internally and to fasten each section to the one next to it. The inside of the hair shaft is called the cortex. By far the largest part of the hair, the cortex occupies 75% to 80% of hair volume and is covered by the cuticle layers. Mechanically, the cortex is the most important part of the hair, and both the tensile strength and elasticity of the hair depend on the cortex. Its many intricate subdivisions are described in this chapter in great detail and supported by many drawings. This chapter also highlights the various differences between Type 1 straight, Caucasian/Oriental hair, Type 2 wavy hair, and Types 3 & 4 curly-to-coily, African-descent hair. The third and innermost section of the hair fiber is the medulla. It is a discontinuous empty space at the very center of the hair, which may even be absent in very fine, thin hair. Its function is not well understood, and more research needs to be devoted to this part of the hair fiber. This chapter also provides various cautionary statements to protect the hair from damage and breakage due to both mechanical and chemical abuses such as excessive brushing and combing or the prolonged application of chemical substances to straighten or lighten the hair.

## References

Breakspear, S., Smith, J. R., & Luengo, G. (2005). Effect of the covalently linked fatty acid 18-MEA on the nanotribology of hair's outermost surface. *Journal of Structural Biology, 149*, 235–242.

Evan, D. J., Leeder, J. D., Rippon, J. A., & Rivett. (1985). *Separation and analysis of surface lipids of the wool fibre.* (Vol. 1, pp. 135–142). Proceedings of the 7th International Wool Textile Research Conference, Tokoyo, Japan.

Feughelman, M. (1997). *Mechanical properties and structure of alpha-keratin fibers: Wool, human hair and related fibers.* Sydney, Australia: University of New South Wales Press

Franbourg, A., & Leroy, F. (2005). Hair structure, function, and physiochemical properties. In Bouillon & Wilkinson (Eds), *The science of hair care* (2nd ed., pp. 1–65). Boca Raton, FL: CRC Taylor & Francis.

Harland, D. P., Vernon, J. A., Woods, J. L., Nagase, S., Itou, T., Kolke, K., ... & Clerens, S. (2018). Intrinsic curvature in wool fibres is determined by the relative length of orthocortical and paracortical cells. *Journal of Experimental Biology, 221*, 1-9.

Hocker, H. (2002). Fiber morphology. In Simpson & Crawshaw (Eds.), *Wool: Science and technology* (pp. 60–79). Cambridge, England: Woodhead.

Jones, L. N., Peet, D. J., Danks, D. M., Negri, A. P., & Rivett, D. E. (1996). Hairs from patients with maple syrup urine disease show a structural defect in the fiber cuticle. The *Journal of Investigative Dermatology, 106*, 461–464.

Kamath, Y. K., Hornby, S. B., & Weigmann, H. D. (1984). Mechanical and fractographic behavior of Negroid hair. *Journal of the Society of Cosmetic Chemists, 35*, 21–43.

Kassenbaum, P. (1981). Morphology and fine structure of hair. In Montagna & Stuttgen (Eds.). *Hair Research* (pp. 52–64). New York, NY: Springer.

Leon, N. H. (1972). Structural aspects of keratin fibers. *Journal of the Society of Cosmetic Chemists, 23*, 427–445.

Nagase, S., Tsuchiya, M., Matsui, T., Shibuichi, S., Tsujimura, H., Satoh, N., & Tsujii, K. (2008). Characterization of curved hair of Japanese women with reference to internal structures and amino acid composition. *Journal of Cosmetic Science, 59*, 317–332.

Parry, D. A. D, & Steinert, P. M. (1999). Intermediate filaments: Molecular architecture, assembly, dynamics and polymorphism. *Quaterly Review of Biophysics, 32*, 99–187.

Robbins, C. R. (2002). *Chemical and physical behavior of human hair* (4th ed.). New York, NY: Springer.

Robbins, C. R. (2009). The cell membrane complex: Three related but different cellular cohesion components of mammalian hair fibers. *Journal of Cosmetic Science, 60*, 437–465.

Rogers, M. A., Langbein, L., Praetzel-Wunder, S., Winter, H., & Schweizer, J. (2006). Human hair keratin-associated proteins (KAPs). *International review of cytology, 251,* 209-263.

Shimomura, Y., & Ito, M. (2005). Human hair keratin-associated proteins. In *Journal of Investigative Dermatology Symposium Proceedings, 10*(3), 230-233.

Swift, J. A. (1999). Human hair cuticle: Biologically conspired to the owner's advantage. *Journal of Cosmetic Science, 50,* 23–45.

Swift, J. A. (2000). Letter to the editor: The cuticle controls bending stiffness of hair. *Journal of Cosmetic Science, 51,* 37–38.

Syed, A. N., Kuhajda, A., Ayoub, H., Ahmad, K., & Frank, E. M 1995, October). African-American hair: Its physical properties and differences relative to Caucasian hair. *Cosmetics & Toiletries Magazine, 110,* 39–48.

Syed, A. N., Ventura, T., & Syed, M. N. (2013). Hair ethnicity and ellipticity: A preliminary study. *Cosmetics & Toiletries Magazine, 128*(4), 250–259.

Wortmann, F. J., & Kure, N. (1994). Effects of the cuticle on the permanent wave set of human hair. *Journal of the Society of Cosmetic Chemists, 45,* 149–158.

# CHAPTER 3

# Hair Textures & Their Properties

Wavy, curly, and coily hair is found all over the world. Historically, hair shape was described by ethnicity/race. For example, slightly wavy to wavy hair is quite prevalent among the Caucasian race in Central American countries, the Middle East, Southern Europe, and South-East Asia. Curly-to-coily hair is found in the United States of America among African-Americans; Puerto Ricans; Cuban-Americans; and Caribbean-Americans, including inhabitants of the Dominican Republic, and other ethnicities. Recently Japanese women, who have commonly been associated with having straight hair, surprisingly displayed a small degree of hair fiber curvature where 47% of Japanese women had slightly wavy to frizzy hair (Nagase et al., 2008, p. 317). Thus, given human migratory patterns over the past few centuries, racial and ethnic descriptions of hair type have become relatively inaccurate and outdated.

It is, therefore, with the intention of finding more objective descriptions of hair shape that attempts have been made to categorize and subcatergorize hair into various types, rather than to describe them by alluding to nationality or ethnic background. Perhaps the most successful attempt at doing this was by renowned hair stylist Andre Walker (1997), who styled the hair of many celebrities, including that of Oprah Winfrey

(p. 24). Walker's classification of hair types was the beginning of hair descriptions in terms of hair waviness or curliness. He described Type 1 as straight hair and classified the next three types of hair on the basis of the degree of curliness where Type 2 was wavy hair, Type 3 was curly hair, and Type 4 was coily hair. Interesting here was that Type 1 had zero waves and was very straight, while the degree of curliness kept increasing from Type 2 to Type 4 hair. Walker further divided each hair type into three subtypes, based on the hair diameter from fine, to medium, to coarse for Type 1 hair. For example, Type 1A was straight hair with a small diameter (fine), Type 1B was straight hair with a medium diameter, and Type 1C was straight hair with a large hair diameter (coarse). This subcategorization was also carried out for Type 2 and Type 3 hair, but on the basis of waviness and not in terms of fineness or coarseness of the hair. Walker divided Type 4 hair into two categories, namely, 4A and 4B, depending upon the hair thickness, which again was based on fiber diameter. Walker did not depict the properties of these hair types based on fiber physics or other basic hair properties as they relate to the physical and chemical properties of hair; neither did he draw a Periodic Table of Hair Straightness/Curliness, with these properties on a continuum. Therefore, this author has devised a modified Periodic Table of Global Textures (**Figures 3.1-3.4**), based on the degree of curl in the hair fiber and the properties of these hair types, explored with the use of scientific techniques.

## Type 1 (Straight) Textures

Type 1 hair, visually depicted in **Figure 3.1**, is completely straight in shape. Caucasian, Northern European, Oriental/Mongoloid, and American-Indian (Native American) hair normally fall into the Type 1 category. There is no wave pattern in this hair type, neither in the wet nor dry state. This hair type possesses a great deal of moisture, strength, elasticity, shine, and smoothness. It also exhibits the lowest degree of porosity and ellipticity. Type 1 hair has the least amount of body and tends to be limp, especially when compared to Types 2, 3, and 4 hair. Type 1 hair can become frizzy when treated with permanent hair colors and hair lighteners due to increased porosity.

# Curly Hair: Structure, Properties, & Care — Chapter 3

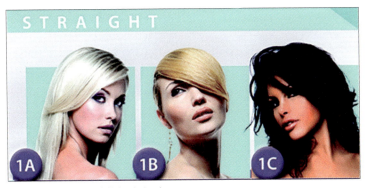

Figure 3.1. Type 1 (straight) hair textures.

## Type 2 (Wavy) Textures

Type 2 hair, visually depicted in **Figure 3.2**, exhibits some degree of waviness. Type 2A hair has the lowest degree of waviness in the wet state; it actually appears straight upon wetting. There is a slight degree of waviness in the dry stage. The curvature of this hair is small. Type 2B hair shows medium waviness, in both wet and dry states. Type 2C hair exhibits more waviness and higher curvature than Type 2B hair.

Type 2 hair possesses high levels of moisture, elasticity, strength, shine, and smoothness, just like Type 1 hair, but it is slightly more elliptical. This hair type also exhibits lower porosity. Type 2 hair is more prone to frizziness and has more body than Type 1 hair. Type 2 hair is prevalent in North America, Latin America, Europe, the Middle East, Southeast Asia, East Asia, and North Africa.

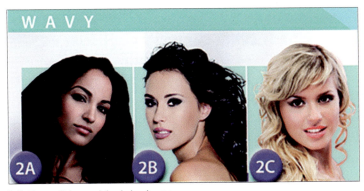

Figure 3.2. Type 2 (wavy) hair textures.

## Type 3 (Curly) Textures

Type 3 hair, visually depicted in **Figure 3.3**, exhibits a high degree of waviness to curliness. Type 3A hair has pronounced waves in both wet and dry states. The degree of wave increases further in Type 3B hair, and it turns to curliness in Type 3C. The curvature of the hair continues to increase from Type 3A to 3B to 3C.

Type 3 hair has significantly less moisture, elasticity, strength, shine, and smoothness when compared to Types 1 and 2 hair. Type 3 hair is significantly more elliptical in shape, exhibits higher porosity, is more prone to frizziness, and has more body than Types 1 and 2 hair. Type 3 hair is prevalent in Latin America (Brazil), the Caribbean, Southern Europe, the Middle East, and North Africa. A significant number of African-American and African-descent individuals possess Type 3C hair.

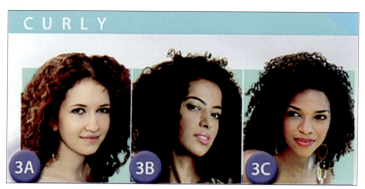

Figure 3.3. Type 3 (curly) hair textures.

## Type 4 (Tightly Curled/Coily) Textures

Type 4 hair, visually depicted in **Figure 3.4**, exhibits a high degree of curliness to coiliness. Type 4A hair has pronounced curls and coils in both the wet and dry states. The coiliness increases further in the case of Types 4B and 4C hair. Type 4C hair becomes tightly coily. The curvature of hair increases to a maximum from Type 3 to Type 4. Upon wetting this hair type, it becomes very coily and shrinks in length.

Type 4 hair has the least amount of moisture, elasticity, strength, shine, and smoothness when compared to Types 1, 2, and 3 hair. Type 4 hair is also highly elliptical. This type of hair further exhibits a high degree of porosity. Type 4 hair has a high amount of body as compared to Types 1, 2, and 3 hair. This hair type is more prone to frizziness in comparison to Types 1, 2, and 3 hair. Type 4 hair is prevalent in the United States (among African-descent individuals), the Caribbean, Northeastern Brazil, and Africa.

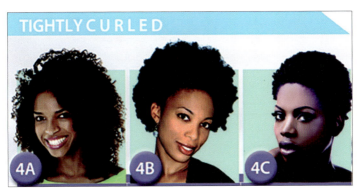

**Figure 3.4.** Type 4 (coily) hair textures.

## Qualitative & Directional Relationship of Hair Type & Hair Properties

The directional relationship, determined qualitatively, between hair type and the hair properties of waviness, porosity, ellipticity, body, frizziness, hair shrinkage, and scalp dryness are shown in **Figure 3.5**.

As can be seen in **Figure 3.5**, waviness, porosity, ellipticity, hair body, hair frizziness, hair shrinkage, and scalp dryness increase from Type 1 to Type 4 hair.

The qualitative or directional relationship of hair type and the amount of moisture, fiber strength/elasticity, ease of combing, shine, and fiber smoothness are shown in **Figure 3.6**. As can be seen in **Figure 3.6**, the amount of moisture, fiber strength/elasticity, ease of combing, shine, and fiber smoothness decrease from Type 1 to Type 4 hair.

A quantitative comparison of some of these properties between Type 1 and Type 4 hair can be found in **Table 3.1**.

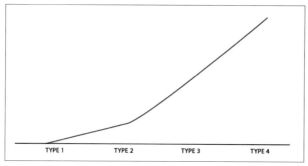

**Figure 3.5.** The directional (qualitative) relationship of hair type to hair waviness, porosity, ellipticity, body, frizziness, and scalp dryness.

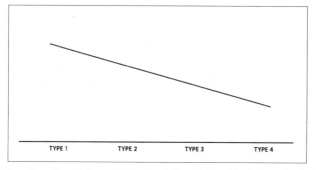

**Figure 3.6.** The directional (qualitative) relationship of hair type to hair moisture, strength/elasticity, ease of combing, shine, and fiber smoothenss.

## Combing Type 3 & Type 4 Hair

One fundamental grooming practice in hair care is combing the hair in both the wet and the dry state. Most consumers comb their hair on a regular basis. The ease of combing one's hair is a very common observation made by consumers of all hair types. Type 1 hair is straight in its configuration and thus very easy to comb. However, the hair becomes more difficult to comb as the degree of wave and curl increases. Type 2 hair is slightly more difficult to comb than Type 1 hair. Type 3 hair is more difficult to comb than Types 1 and 2 hair. Type 4 hair is more difficult to comb than Types 1, 2 and 3 hair.

**Figure 3.7 (A)** shows the total combing energy required to comb Type 1 (straight, Caucasian) hair vs Type 4 (curly/coily, African-Amerian) hair in both the wet and dry states. It was observed that Type 4 wet hair

**TABLE 3.1** *Quantitative Measurements of Hair Properties of Type 1 & Type 4*

| PROPERTIES | TYPE 1<br>CAUCASIAN HAIR | TYPE 4<br>AFRICAN-DESCENT HAIR |
|---|---|---|
| **EASE OF WET COMBING**<br>(Syed & Syed, 2017, p. 20) | Very Easy | 23 times more difficult |
| **EASE OF DRY COMBING**<br>(Syed & Syed, 2017, p. 20) | Very Easy | 32 times more difficult |
| **EASE OF DISENTAGLING – WET**<br>(Syed & Syed, 2017. p. 20) | Very Easy | 19 times more difficult |
| **EASE OF DISENTAGLING – DRY**<br>(Syed & Syed, 2017. p. 20) | Very Easy | 20 times more difficult |
| **ELASTICITY OF WET FIBERS AT 0.50% EXTENSION**<br>(Syed & Syed, 2017, p. 17) | 1.92 times stronger | Very Weak |
| **TENSILE STRENGTH – WET**<br>(Syed et al., 1995, p. 44) | 1.47 times stronger | Very Weak |
| **TENSILE STRENGTH – DRY**<br>(Syed et al., 1995, p. 44) | 1.26 times stronger | Very Weak |
| **SHAPE** | Close to Cylindrical<br>Ellipticity is 1.0 to 1.4 | Oval and Irregular<br>Ellipticity is 1.0 to 3.2 |
| **ELLIPTICITY VARIANCE WITHIN A FIBER**<br>(Syed & Syed, 2017. p. 11) | 2.0% | 22.0% |
| **CUTICLE LAYERS**<br>(Leon, 1972, p. 435) | 6 - 10 Layers | 2 Layers: Outer Crimp<br>6-10 Layers: Inner Crimp |
| **POROSITY** | Significantly Lower | Significantly Higher |
| **HAIR GROWTH**<br>(Loussouarn, 2001, p. 294 Africans)<br>(Lewallen et al., 2016, p.-African American) | Average ± SE<br>5.69 ± 0.12 inch/year<br>4.74 ± 0.04 inch per year | Average ± SE<br>3.68 ± 0.01 inch/year<br>3.72 ± 0.04 inches per year |
| **STATIC ELECTRICITY**<br>(Syed et al., 1995, p. 44) | Very Low | Very High & With Negative Sign |
| **SHINE** | Significantly more | Significantly less |
| **MOISTURE CONTENTS OF DRY HAIR AT**<br>**40% RELATIVE HUMIDITY:**<br>**70% RELATIVE HUMIDITY:**<br>(Syed et al., 2019, p. 4) | High<br>High | 19% Lower<br>14% Lower |
| **MOISTURE CONTENTS OF SCALP** | More | Less |
| **TRANSEPIDERMAL WATER LOSS OF THE SCALP (TEWL)** | Less | More |
| **RATIO OF TWISTS** | 1.0 | 3.67 |

requires 23 times more force to comb than Type 1 wet hair (Syed & Syed, 2017, p. 20). Similarly, Type 4 dry hair requires 32 times more combing energy than Type 1 dry hair. It is very difficult to detangle Type 4 hair as compared to Type 1 hair. **Figure 3.7 (B)** shows the total force, measured as the maximum peak load, required to detangle Type 1 hair vs Type 4 hair

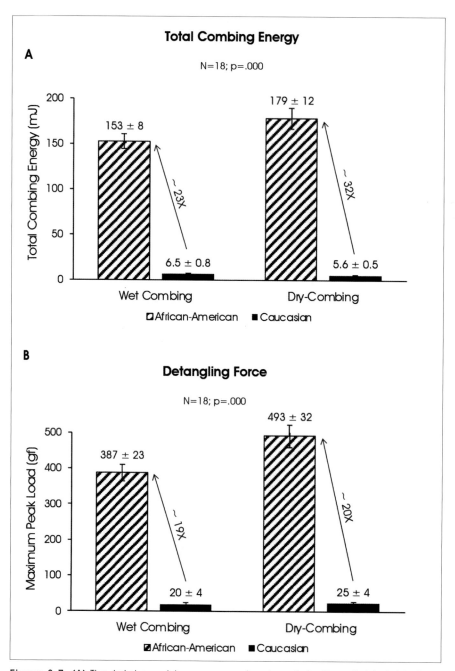

Figure 3.7. **(A)** The total combing energy of wet and dry Type 1 (straight, Caucasian) and Type 4 (curly/coily, African-American) hair. **(B)** The force (maximum peak load) required to detangle Type 1 (straight, Caucasian) and Type 4 (curly/coily, African-American) hair in the wet and dry states.

in both the wet and dry states. The force required to detangle Type 4 hair in the wet state is 19 times higher than the force required for Type 1 hair. The force required to detangle Type 4 dry hair is 20 times greater than that required for Type 1 dry hair.

## Hair Elasticity Comparison of Type 1 & Type 4 Hair

Elasticity is a measure of fiber strength at low strain values. For example, in our study elasticity was measured at 0.5% strain. It is important to measure fiber strength at low strain as these strains are representative of the everyday manipulation of hair fibers through pulling, twisting, or simply running your fingers through your hair.

**Figure 3.8** shows the wet fiber elasticity of Type 1 (straight, Caucasian) hair vs Type 4 (curly/coily, African-descent) hair. Wet fiber elasticity of Type 1 hair is 65.75 ± 1.51 g/denier (average ± se), and the wet fiber elasticity of Type 4 hair is 34.24 ± 1.17 g/denier, as shown in **Figure 3.8**. Type 1 hair is 1.92 times stronger than Type 4 hair (Syed & Syed, 2017, p. 16). Therefore, as the hair becomes curlier/coilier, its elasticity and strength decreases. It is, therefore, incumbent upon hair care experts and consumers alike to avoid extra manipulation of curly/coily hair to avoid

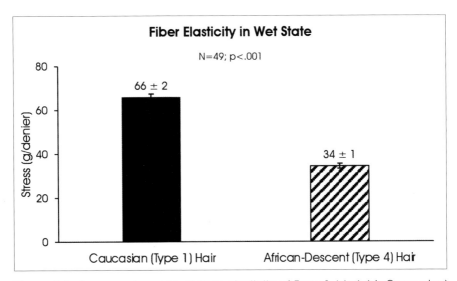

Figure 3.8. A comparison of wet fiber elasticity of Type 1 (straight, Caucasian) and Type 4 (curly/coily, African-descent) hair at 0.5% strain.

damage and hair breakage.

## Shape of Wavy and Curly/Coily Hair

Type 1 hair is straight in its shape, while Types 2, 3, and 4 hair have some degree of curl. Type 2 hair is wavy in shape. Type 3 hair is curly in shape and Type 4 hair is curly to coily in shape. The degree of curl increases from Types 2A, B, and C to Types 3A and 3B. From Type 3C to Type 4C, the hair fiber changes its shape from curly to coily with many twists. The internal physical and chemical properties of the fiber structure also change from Type 1 to Types 2, 3, and 4.

**Figure 3.9** shows photographs of Type 1 to Type 4 hair fibers. Type 1 hair is cylindrical, whereas Type 2 hair has a slight wave in the fibers. Types 3A and 3B are wavier; Type 3C is very curly with a shorter wave diameter; and Types 4A, B, and C are springlike coils. In Type 4 hair, the coils become tighter, and they shrink from Type 4A to 4C.

The three-dimensional shape of Type 1 hair is quite cylindrical, whereas Types 2, 3, and 4 are increasingly ovoid (oval) in shape. The ovality of hair fibers is measured in terms of their ellipticity. Ellipticity is defined as the ratio between major axis and minor axis of a hair fiber. A perfect cylinder has an ellipticity of 1.0, whereas oval shapes have ellipticities of more than 1. The ellipticity of Type 1 hair fibers is approximately 1.0-1.4, and the ellipticity of curly hair is ~ 1.895 (Kamath et al., 1984, p. 25). The ellipticity of wavy and curly hair varies along the hair shaft from 1.0-3.2, giving wavy/curly hair a unique feature (Syed & Ventura, 2013, p. 258). The shapes of Type 1 and Type 4 hair, in terms of their ellipticity, are shown in **Figure 3.10**.

Type 1 and Type 2 hair fibers are smooth because of low ellipticity, whereas Type 3 and Type 4 hair fibers are not smooth due to high ellipticity and high variation in ellipticity along the hair shaft. The variation in ellipticity within each fiber was determined by the coefficient of variation of ellipticity, which was 2.0% for Type 1 hair and 22.0% for Type 4 hair (Syed & Syed, 2017, p. 11).

*Curly Hair: Structure, Properties, & Care* **Chapter 3**

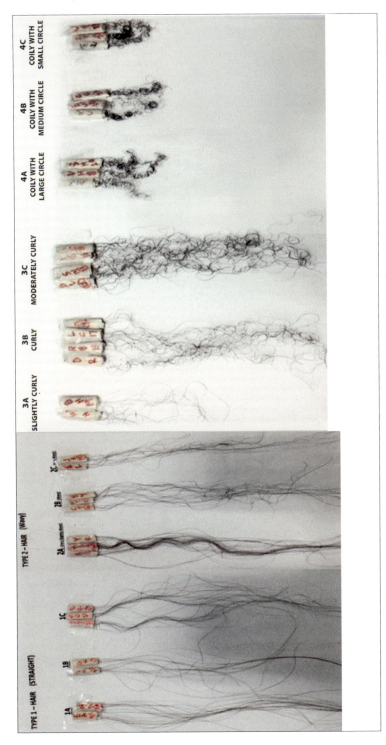

**Figure 3.9.** Real human hair fibers matched to hair type. Type 1 is straight hair, Type 2 is wavy hair, Type 3 is curly hair and Type 4 is coily hair. The shape of the hair in terms of straightness, waviness, curliness, and coiliness are depicted in these photographs. As the degree of curliness in the hair fibers increases, the hair fibers appear to be shorter in length.

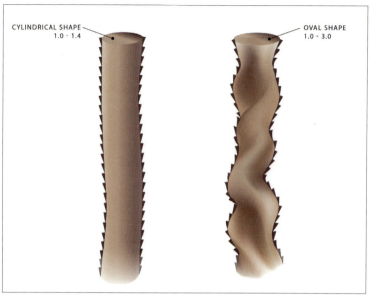

Figure 3.10. Ellipticity of Type 1 (left) and Type 4 (right) hair compared: Type 1 hair is almost cylindrical whereas Type 4 hair is elliptical; The ellipticity of Type 4 hair changes from point to point along the hair shaft, leading to the lowest degree of smoothness when compared to other hair types.

## Relationship of Cortical Cells & the Shape of Hair

Hair fibers are made of outer cuticle layers and inner cortical cells. These cortical cells are of two distinct shapes and are called para and ortho (Mercer, 1953, p. 394), shown in **Figure 3.11**. Paracortical cells are spindle-shaped cells, and orthocortical cells are also spindle shaped but longer.

The amount of para- vs orthocortical cells, and their packing pattern determines the final shape of the hair fiber. **Figure 3.12** shows

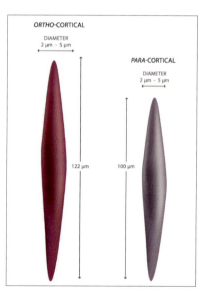

Figure 3.11. Illustration of para and orthocortical cells. Orthocortical cells are longer.

# Curly Hair: Structure, Properties, & Care — Chapter 3

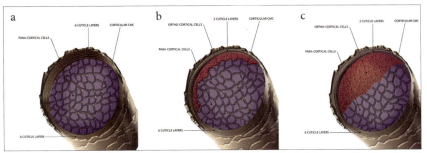

Figure 3.12. (a) Type 1, straight hair, shows the presence of paracortical cells only; (b) Type 2 and Types 3A and 3B show the presence of mostly paracortical cells and 1–3 rows of orthocortical cells; (c) Type 3C and Type 4 show approximately equal rows of paracortical cells and orthocortical cells.

the different packing composition and arrangements in the cortex of (a) Type 1 hair, (b) Type 2 and Type 3A and Type 3B, and (c) Type 3C and Type 4 hair. Type 1 hair is composed of only paracortical cells, arranged hexagonally inside the cortex, which is the reason why the fiber has a completely straight shape (Feughelman, 1997, p. 6). Type 2 and up to Type 3B, hair is composed of a few rows (1–3) of orthocortical cells; the rest is composed of paracortical cells. The cortex of Type 3C to Type 4C hair contains approximately equal rows of orthocortical and paracortical cells that face each other. In the case of wavy/curly, curly, and coily hair, the orthocortical cells are arranged in a whorllike pattern in the cortex. This packing pattern of orthocortical cells is responsible for the wavy and coily shape of the fibers. The increasing amount of orthcortical cells in the cortex changes hair from straight to wavy, to curly, to coily. The higher the number of orthocortical cells in the cortex, the curlier the hair becomes.

In wavy or curly/coily hair, the paracortical cells are on the inside of the crimp and the orthocortical cells are on the outside of the crimp. The shape of wavy or curly/coily hair with respect to the position of ortho- and paracortical cells is shown in **Figure 3.13**.

## The Number of Cuticle Layers in Various Hair Types

The literature generated by hairstylists and consumers is not very clear regarding the number of cuticles in wavy/curly hair. Authors generally assume that the same number of cuticles are present in wavy/

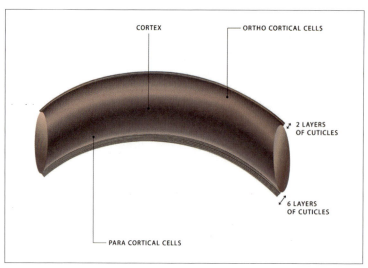

**Figure 3.13.** The orthocortical cells are on the outer side of the crimp; the paracortical cells are on the inner side of the crimp. The inner side of the crimp (the paracortex) in a curly hair has 6 cuticle layers, while the outer side of the crimp in curly hair (the orthocortex) has only 2 layers of cuticles.

curly hair as in straight hair. Hairstylists and consumers in the wavy/curly hair segment of the population believe that the cuticles in their hair merely stand up more than they do for individuals with straight hair. They may not realize that a wavy or curly hair fiber exhibits differing numbers of cuticle layers on the inner and outer crimp of a hair fiber and that this trend continues along the length of the fiber. This condition of varying cuticle layers on the inner and outer sides of a curly hair along the hair length is shown in **Figure 3.13**.

This feature of varying cuticle layers on the inner and outer sides of the hair shaft is also responsible for the greater hair porosity in individuals with curly hair. Straight hair exhibits significantly lower porosity than curly hair because of the presence of 6 to 10 cuticle layers placed in a uniform manner along the hair shaft.

## Porosity of Types 1, 2, 3, & 4 Hair

Porosity is a measure of the capacity of a hair fiber to absorb and retain liquids and moisture. Hair that absorbs more liquid or moisture has

Curly Hair: Structure, Properties, & Care                    **Chapter 3**

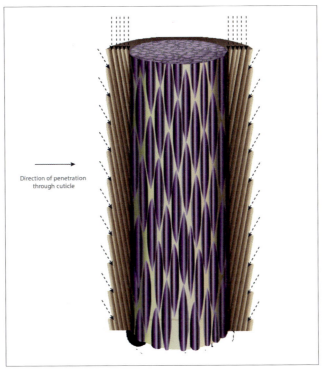

**Figure 3.14.** Schematic of the mechanism of water absorption by the hair cortex through the channels between cuticle layers.

a higher porosity and vice versa. The term hair porosity refers to the small openings and channels within the cuticles (**Figure 3.14**) that allow gases, liquids, or microscopic particles to pass into the cortex and the degree of weight retention of these molecules in the hair. When hair fibers are immersed in water, they absorb different quantities of water or moisture. If the fibers have damaged or fewer cuticle layers, the hair cortex will absorb more moisture because of high porosity. If the fiber contains more cuticle layers that are healthy, the hair will absorb less water—it has low porosity.

Methods such as the Sink Test and the Liquid Retention Test are used to measure hair fiber porosity. The Sink Test is based on placing hair fibers on the surface of a glass full of water and noting the time it takes for the fibers to sink to the bottom of the glass. If the fibers float for a long period of time, they have low porosity, but if they sink fast, they have high porosity, as shown in **Figure 3.15**. The Sink Test is convenient for a consumer to perform at home but it is only a qualitative test, as it does not offer any quantitative porosity numbers. To make the Sink Test quantitatively discriminating will require some efforts to streamline the method.

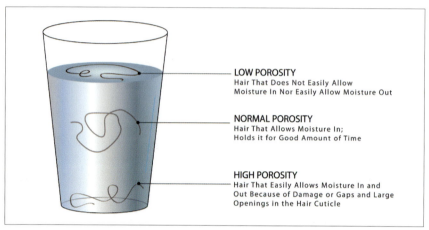

Figure 3.15. Illustration of the Sink Test set-up for qualitatively assessing porosity. The time it takes to sink hair fibers is determined by the porosity of the hair.

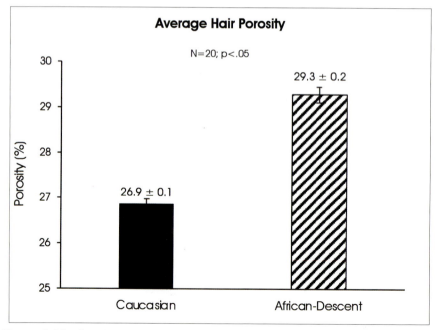

Figure 3.16. Graph comparing the porosity (%) of Caucasian (Type 1) and African-descent (Types 3 and 4) hair.

The Valko and Barnett (1952) method is a more accurate, scientific procedure for measuring porosity. It was subsequently revised by Menkart et al. (1966) and has been used extensively by the scientific community to determine the porosity of hair (Syed & Ayoub, 2002, p. 58). With this method, the hair fibers are first cleansed with a nonconditioning shampoo and rinsed extensively with water. The fibers are then towel blotted and dried at room temperature, until dry. A bundle of 0.50 g hair sample is prepared and equilibrated at 65% RH for 24 hours. The hair fibers are then weighed accurately at 65% RH. These hair fibers are then immersed in deionized water for 30 minutes. Then, the fibers are removed from the water and spun in a centrifuge at 7200 RPM, for 10 minutes. After centrifuging the fibers, they are weighed again, and the weight gain of the fibers is calculated. The results are shown in **Figure 3.16** where the average porosity of Caucasian hair was found to be 26.87 ± 0.10 (average ± se), and the porosity of African-American fibers was found to be 29.28 ± 0.17, which is significantly higher than Caucasian hair porosity at $p < .05$.

The porosity data for both hair types were analyzed for number of groups within each category. The porosity differences in Caucasian hair were very small, and all data fell into one group. The porosity data from 20 African-American individuals fell in several groups, suggesting that the hair porosity of African-American individuals has greater variance and can be categorized into low, medium, and high porosity (Syed & Syed, 2017, p. 27).

## Comparing the Hair Growth of Caucasian & African-Descent Individuals

Hair growth seems to have more importance in the African-American community, considering that many individuals in this community complain that their hair does not grow fast enough. Many different views are expressed in this community, ranging from low hair growth rate to equal hair growth rate. Many times, it is quoted that the hair growth rate of Caucasians is approximately 1 inch per 2 months, or 6 inches per year. The growth rate of hair of African-descent individuals has been quantified by two different studies to date: the Loussouarn study and the Lewallen study. These studies answer many questions related to hair growth for different ethnicities, as well as dispel some myths. Hair growth will be discussed in detail in Chapter 4 but we will briefly touch upon it here.

The study by Loussouarn (2001) compared the hair growth of Africans from Central and Western Africa with that of Caucasians. The participants were both men and women, ranging in age from 17 to 37 years. The study examined hair density, telogen percentage, and growth rate. The author studied the vertex, temporal, and occipital areas of the head.

**Hair density.** Hair density varied from 90 to 290 hairs per square centimeter, the hair count at the vertex was higher than in other areas, and no significant differences in growth rate were found between or among men and women. The average hair density among men and women was found to be 190 ± 40 hairs per square centimeter.

**Telogen.** Telogen is the resting phase of the hair growth cycle. It follows the anagen phase, during which the hair grows significantly. Normally, 90% of the hair fibers on a person's head are in the anagen phase. As the telogen phase follows the anagen phase, approximately 5% of hairs find themselves in the telogen phase at any given time. After the telogen phase, the hair enters the exogen phase, in which hair sheds from the scalp during combing and hairstyling. After the exogen phase, the hair follicle enters the anagen phase once more and produces a new hair in the place of the lost hair. This cycling through the anagen, telogen, and exogen phases continues as long as the hair follicle is alive.

There were large variations from 2% to 46% in the telogen phases of the study participants, where the temporal area, especially among men, showed the highest telogen phase percentage. The average telogen phase for Africans was found to be 18 ± 9%, as compared to 14 ± 11% for Caucasians.

**Growth rate.** The average growth rate of hair among Africans was 256 (μm) microns per day, as compared to 396 μm per day for Caucasians.

Loussouarn (2001) further compared these data with data from Caucasian individuals of similar age. The findings are listed in **Table 3.2**, where the data are converted from centimeters to inches for American readers.

As shown in **Table 3.2**, Caucasian hair grows ~5.6906 inches per year, which is close to the general belief in consumer circles, whereas African hair grows at a significantly slower rate of ~3.6787 inches per year.

Table 3.2 *Comparison of Hair Density, Telogen Hairs, and Growth Rate Between Africans and Caucasians of Similar Age*

| Property | Africans | Caucasians |
|---|---|---|
| Density (hairs/square inch) | 1226 ± 258 | 1465 ± 355 |
| Telogen Hairs (%) | 18 ± 9 | 14 ± 11 |
| Rate of Hair Growth (inches/year) | 3.6787 | 5.6906 |

Note: All reported values are averages. Telogen is the resting phase in the hair growth cycle. Averages reported by Loussouarn (2001).

Loussouarn (2001) concluded that African-descent hair grows 35% slower than Caucasian hair, the density of African-descent hair per square inch is 16% lower than that of Caucasian hair, and hairs of African-descent individuals stay 22% longer in the telogen phase than hairs of Caucasians, which would explain the slow rate of growth of African-descent hair. It is important to note that this study was conducted with individuals from Central and Western Africa, and results may vary if the tests are replicated with African-Americans because of the mixing of races between African Americans and Caucasian Americans over the last few centuries.

## Static Charge on African-American Hair

Static charge on hair fibers is measured after combing the hair. Untreated African-descent hair develops a highly negative electrostatic charge (-25.4 KV/m). Upon relaxing African-descent hair with alkali metal hydroxide creams, the charge changes to +25.9 KV/meter. In contrast, Caucasian hair develops a very low positive electrostatic charge of +6.6 KV/m (Syed, 2006, p. 539). The relatively high negative charge acquired by dry African-descent hair during combing may be due to the high degree of pulling force required to pass the comb through the mass of entangled hair fibers and due to the lower amount of 18-MEA on curly/coily hair fiber surfaces (Breakspear et al., 2005, p. 241). The combing of untreated or chemically straightened African-descent hair develops a significantly higher electrostatic charge than Caucasian hair. This relatively high electrostatic charge produces a "balloon effect" that contributes to a greater degree of hair unmanageability (Morton & Hearle, 1986, p. 535).

## Hair Shine

Type 4 (curly/coily, African-descent) hair possesses high curvature and is also considerably more twisted than its counterpart, Type 1 (straight, Caucasian) hair. The cuticles are raised in Type 4 hair and thus do not reflect light as readily as the ones of Type 1 hair.

## Moisture Content of Type 1 & Type 4 Hair

Type 1 hair seems to hold more moisture than Type 3 and Type 4 hair. Very few studies, if any, seem to have referred to the moisture in Type 4 hair. New methods are available now to conduct moisture-content studies using a microwave resonance technique. This technique has been used to compare and contrast the moisture content of Type 1 and Type 4 hair. The African-descent hair samples were taken from a single human head, and their validity was certified. It is important to note that the data

Table 3.3 *Moisture Content of Type 1 and Type 4 Hair as a Function of Relative Humidity*

| Relative Humidity | Moisture Content (%) | | Percent Difference |
|---|---|---|---|
| | Type 1 Hair | Type 4 Hair | |
| 40% | 8.57 ± 0.06 | 6.90 ± 0.06 | < 19.49% |
| 70% | 12.14 ± 0.06 | 10.50 ± 0.07 | < 3.51% |

Average and standard error reported. $p < .05$; $N=11$

were collected from a sample provided by only one African-American individual. More extensive studies will need to be conducted using hair samples from many African-American individuals. The moisture content data of Type 1 and Type 4 hair are based on a study by Syed and Mathew (2019) and shown in **Table 3.3**. These data are also depicted in **Figure 3.17**.

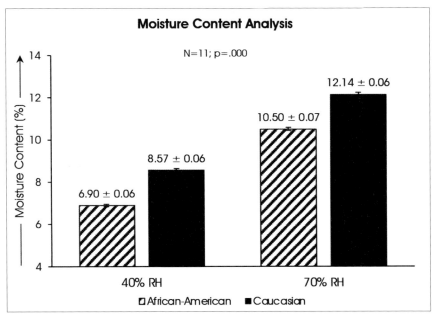

Figure 3.17. Moisture content of Type 4 (curly/coily, African-American) hair and Type 1 (straight, Caucasian) hair at 40% and 70% relative humidity (RH).

**Table 3.3** and **Figure 3.17** clearly show that Type 4 (curly/coily, African-American) hair has 19.49% less moisture at 40% RH, and 13.51% less moisture at 70% RH than Type 1 (straight, Caucasian) hair. This lack of moisture in Type 4 hair is significant. It is, therefore, imperative that treatment products incorporate a high degree of moisture for Type 4 hair in order to enhance such hair properties as "anti-dry" feel and strength.

## References

Breakspear, S., Smith, J. R., & Luengo, G. (2005). Effect of the covalently linked fatty acid 18-MEA on the nanotribology of hair's outermost surface. Journal of Structural Biology, 149, 235–242.

Feughelman, M. (1997). Mechanical properties and structure of alpha-keratin fibers: Wool, human hair and related fibers. Sydney, Australia: University of New South Wales Press.

Kamath, Y. K., Hornby, S. B., & Weigmann, H. D. (1984). Mechanical and fractographic behavior of Negroid hair. Journal of the Society of Cosmetic Chemists, 35, 21–43.

Leon, N. H. (1972). Structural aspects of keratin fibers. Journal of the Society of Cosmetic Chemists, 23, 427–445.

Loussouarn, G. (2001). African hair growth parameters. British Journal of Dermatology, 145, 294–297.

Menkart, J., Wolfram, L. J., & Mao, I. (1966). Caucasian hair, Negro hair, and wool: Similarities and differences. Journal of the Society of Cosmetic Chemists, 17, 769–787.

Mercer, E. H. (1953). The heterogeneity of the keratin fibers. Textile Research Journal, 23(6), 388–397.

Morton, W. E., & Hearle, J. W. S. (1986). Physical properties of textile fibres. Manchester, UK: The Textile Institute.

Nagase, S., Tsuchiya, M., Matsui, T., Shibuichi, S., Tsujimura, H., Satoh, N., . . . & Tsujii, K. (2008). Characterization of curved hair of Japanese women with reference to internal structures and amino acid composition. Journal of Cosmetic Science, 59, 317–332.

Syed, A. N. (2006). Hair straightening. In M. Schlossman (Ed.), The chemistry and manufacture of cosmetics (Vol. II, pp. 535–557). Carol Stream, IL: Allured Publishing.

Syed, A. N., & Ayoub, H. (2002). Correlating porosity and tensile strength of chemically modified hair. Cosmetics & Toiletries Magazine, 117(11), 57–64.

Syed, A. N., & Syed, M. N. (2017). Textured hair: Its characteristics and comparison against nontextured hair. SCC Symposium, October 12, 2017, New York, NY.

Syed, A. N., Kuhajda, A., Ayoub, H., Ahmad, K., & Frank, E. M. (1995, October). African-American hair: Its physical properties and differences relative to Caucasian hair. Cosmetics & Toiletries Magazine, 110, 39–48.

Syed, A. N., Mathew, J., & Kazmi, H. (2018). Counting twists in African-American and Caucasian Hair. Avlon® Research Center. Avlon® R & D Report No. 2018-85, 1-6.

Syed, A. N., Mathew, J., & Kazmi, H. (2019). Comparison of moisture contents of hair etween

African-Decent (Type 4) hair and Caucasian (Type 1) hair. Avlon˚ Research Center. Unpublished R & D Report No. 2019-69, 1–5.

Syed, A. N., Ventura, T., & Syed, M. N. (2013). Hair ethnicity and ellipticity: A preliminary study. Cosmetics & Toiletries Magazine, 128(4), 250–259.

Valko, E. I., & Barnett, G. (1952). A study of the swelling of the hair in mixed aqueous solvents. Journal of Society of Cosmetic Chemists, 3, 108–117.

Walker, A. (1997). Andre talks hair. New York, NY: Simon & Schuster.

# CHAPTER 4

# Scalp & Hair Growth
## Hair Loss & Remedies

### The Scalp

According to the popular saying, "the Scalp is the Mother of All Hair," it is implied that the scalp is somewhat different from the rest of the human skin: It grows hair more actively, and it is responsible for the appealing appearance of a woman or man. A head of hair is part of the beauty of a person, and billions of dollars are spent yearly for growing or grooming the hair on the human scalp. The health of the scalp and its ongoing maintenance are crucial for healthy hair and its growth. It is vital to keep the scalp clean, pH-balanced, moisturized, and free of fungus (dandruff) and itching. Progrowth nutrients must be supplied to the scalp either topically or through daily food intake.

A human head has an average of 100,000 to 150,000 hair fibers (Bernard, 2005, p. 73). The scalp is a unique skin site where itching and external stresses are experienced by 25% to 30% of the human population (Dubief, Mellul, Loussouarn, & Saint-Léger, 2005, p. 129). Itching related to dry scalp and bacteria on the scalp could be even higher, especially among African-descent individuals. Cardin (1998) cited one estimate that pegged the incident of scalp itching due to dandruff at 50% of the general population (p. 193), with its prevalence greater among African-descent individuals.

Another apparent difference in comparing the health of the African-descent scalp with the Caucasian scalp is in the moisture content and the transepidermal water loss (TEWL) of the scalp. Very few studies have been conducted to compare the moisture content and TEWL values of African-descent and Caucasian scalps. One such study was conducted by this author with 25 participants and the results are shown in **Table 4.1**.

Table 4.1 *Moisture and TEWL Comparison of Caucasian vs African-American Scalps*

| Property | Caucasian | African-American | p |
|---|---|---|---|
| Moisture (µS) | 40 ± 3 | 29 ± 2 | 0.008 |
| TEWL (g/m²/hr) | 22.1 ± 0.9 | 28 ± 2 | 0.005 |

Note: Average and standard error values are reported. N=25.

The scalps of African-American individuals were found to have an average moisture of 29 ± 2 microSiemens ($\mu S$) (average ± se). The scalps of Caucasian individuals displayed an average moisture of 40 ± 3 $\mu S$ (Syed, et al., 2022, p. 50). Thus, the scalp of African-American individuals showed 28% less moisture than the scalp of Caucasian individuals ($p = .008$). The average TEWL values of the scalp were 28 ± 2 g/m²/h and 22.1 ± 0.9 g/m²/h for African-Americans and Caucasians, respectively, indicating that the scalps of African-American individuals tended to lose more moisture (27%) and were drier than the scalps of Caucasian individuals ($p = .005$).

## Hair Follicle

**Dermal papilla.** The dermal papilla is a large structure at the base of the hair follicle, located near the center of the bulb. It is ovoid, or pear shaped, as shown in **Figure 4.1**. It plays a major role in the development of the hair follicle during the Anagen, Catagen, and Telogen phases (Robbins, 2002, p. 4). The papilla consists mainly of connective tissue and a capillary loop. Cell division in the papilla is very rare to nonexistent.

Curly Hair: Structure, Properties, & Care    Chapter 4

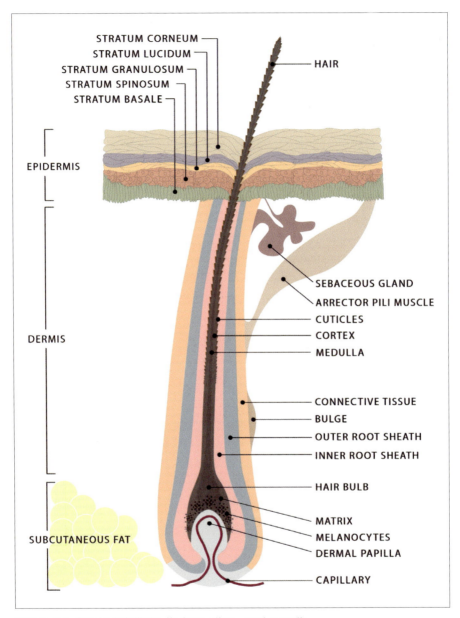

Figure 4.1. The hair follicle, its formation, and growth.

**Hair bulb.** The hair bulb is the lower expanded extremity, which fits like a cap over the hair papilla at the bottom portion of the follicle. The melanocytes exist in the hair bulb and produce hair pigment. The blood vessels deliver nourishment to the hair bulb to grow hair fibers deep within the skin. Biological synthesis and orientation take place at and around the hair bulb. The area around the hair bulb is also called the *zone of cell proliferation and differentiation* (Robbins, 2002, p. 4).

Cell proliferation is the process whereby a cell grows and divides to produce two daughter cells as equal copies. Cell proliferation is responsible for exponential increases in the number of cells (Conlon & Raff, 1999). The proliferated cells change from one cell to another and become differentiated into specialized cells that make up tissues and organs. There are four main tissue types in the human body: epithelial, connective, muscle, and nerve tissue (Light, 2009, p. 20).

**Hair matrix**. The hair matrix exists around the papilla and hair bulb. The structure of hair derives its existence from a single stem cell group called the *matrix of the hair bulb* (Draelos & Pugliese, 2011, p. 44). There are three concentric rings that arise from the matrix of the hair bulb. The three inner rings, from the center outward, are the medulla, cortex, and cuticles. The three outer rings, proceeding from the matrix outward, are the inner root sheath (IRS), the outer root sheath (ORS), and connective tissues.

A collection of epithelial cells is often interspersed with the pigment-producing cells, called *melanocytes*. The division of cells takes place in the hair matrix where the major structures of the hair fiber and the IRS are formed. The hair matrix epithelium is one of the fastest growing cell populations in the human body. These cells are destroyed during chemotherapy or radiotherapy, causing temporary hair loss. The matrix wraps around the papilla, except at the bottom where it is connected to the surrounding connective tissue, which provides access for the capillary. The function of the capillary is to provide blood supply and deliver nutrients for the growth of hair. The centrally located matrical cells of the matrix are responsible for the existence of the IRS. The function of the IRS is to cover the stem of the follicle and protect the bulb and matrix where the hair is growing (Joshi, 2011, p. 57). The IRS is covered by the ORS, which encloses the IRS and the hair shaft. The ORS continues upward to the basal layer of the epidermis. Its role is to protect the hair bulb, the hair shaft, and IRS.

**Arrector pili muscles**. These small muscles are attached to the hair follicle. Their contractions cause the hair to stand on end, creating goose bumps (Cormack, 2001, p. 1). The pressure exerted by the muscles may force the sebum to travel along the hair follicle toward the surface, thereby, protecting the hair against moisture loss.

**Sebaceous glands**. The sebaceous glands are exocrine glands, which secrete an oily or waxy matter, called sebum, to lubricate and waterproof the skin and hair of human beings. These glands are present on the face and scalp, as well as on other parts of the body; the exceptions are the palms of the hands and soles of the feet. The secretion of the sebaceous glands is called *holocrine*, a secretion of dead cells.

**Names of the developing hair fiber**. An unborn baby's hair, from two to eight months during pregnancy, is called *lanugo hair*. Immature hair, which ranges from birth to puberty, is called *villus hair*; it has variable texture. Mature hair, from puberty onward, is called *terminal hair*. The hair follicle, its formation, and growth are depicted in **Figure 4.1**.

## The Shape of Hair

The shape of hair is determined by the hair follicle, and the shape of the follicle depends on the cortical cells it contains. A curly hair follicle is curved because it contains both ortho- and paracortical cells (Thibaut, Barbarat, Leroy, & Bernard, 2007, p. 8), shown in **Figure 4.2** as ortho cortex and para cortex, respectively. A straight hair follicle consists of only paracortical cells. From **Figure 4.2** it can be seen that the lower concave shape of the follicle is due to the orthocortex, and the convex shape of the follicle is due to the paracortex (Hocker, 2002, p. 72). Region 1 contains Type I (acidic) and Type II (basic to neutral) proteins, which are present just above the bulb of the follicle. In Region 2, orthocortical cells contain keratin associated proteins (KAPs) 6, 7, and 8. Region 3 contains KAPs 1, 2, and 3. In the higher area, which is Region 4, the paracortex contains KAP 4, and in the still higher Region 5, cuticles contain KAPs 5 and 10. These KAPs represent the genes of various portions of the follicle.

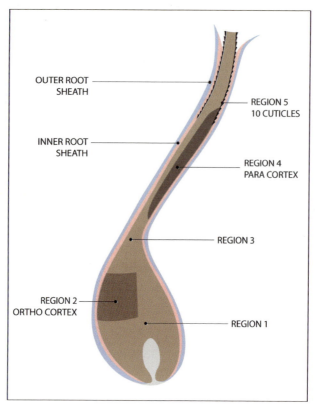

**Figure 4.2.** The shape of a curly hair follicle, depicting ortho- and paracortex and regions that contain different types of KAPs.

Studies revealed that protein hHa8 is accumulated on the concave side of the follicle in a curly/coily hair (Thibaut et al., 2007, p. 9). The concave side of the follicle consists of orthocortex, marked as Region 2, in **Figure 4.2**. In straight hair, protein hHa8 is evenly distributed throughout the follicle.

## Hair Growth

Each hair strand grows for an average of two to six years (Robbins, 2002, p. 9; Thomas, 2005, p. 180). Each follicle can grow 20 hairs sequentially. For Caucasians, the average growth rate is ~0.50 in per month whereas for African-descent individuals, the average growth rate is ~0.30 in per month (Bernard, 2005, p. 73). In one estimate, the average Anagen phase can last from two to seven years (Dhariwala & Ravikumar, 2019, p. 968). A hair strand can grow in length from 12 to 36 in, over two to six years, and, in some exceptional cases, even longer, before it enters a resting phase and, finally, sheds. The follicles decrease in size and number with age.

## The Hair Growth Cycle

Hair growth takes place in three phases, as shown in **Figure 4.3**. The first phase is known as the Anagen phase. There is intense metabolic activity in the hair bulb, and a hair is produced that keeps growing during this phase. The Anagen phase exists up to 90% in the spring and 80% in the late fall (Robbins, 2002, p. 13). About 1% to 5% of hairs transition into the Catagen phase before entering the Telogen phase. The Catagen phase may last from 1 to 3 weeks (Dhariwala & Ravikumar, 2019, p. 967). According to Kligman (1988), 10% of the total number of hairs on a human head are in the Catagen phase at any given time (p. 112). In this phase, the hair fiber stops growing and enters a transition from growth to rest. The hairs that

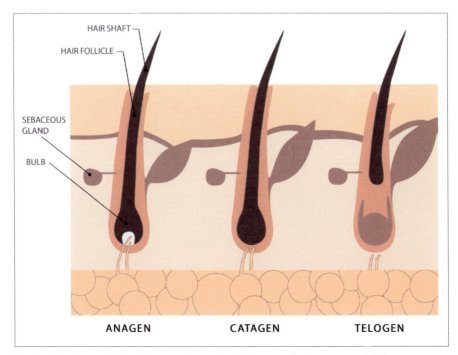

**Figure 4.3.** Three phases of hair growth: Anagen, Catagen, and Telogen.

were in the Catagen (transition) phase enter the third phase, the Telogen phase, where the transitioning hairs enter into a resting state. About 10% to 15% of healthy hair fibers on a human head are generally in the Telogen phase at any given time (Shai et al., 2002, p. 257).

Normally, a human being should lose only 50 to 100 hair fibers in a day during combing (Robbins, 2002, p. 13). If the number of fibers in the Telogen phase increases by more than 10%, excessive hair shedding (>100 fibers/daily) and hair thinning will be observed. Hair fibers in the resting phase will start to fall out of the scalp after a while, which is called the Exogen phase. After the Exogen phase, the hair bulb re-enters the Anagen phase once more, and a new hair starts to grow. A schematic of the normal hair growth cycle that depicts various hair growth stages, their durations, and percentages is shown in **Figure 4.4**.

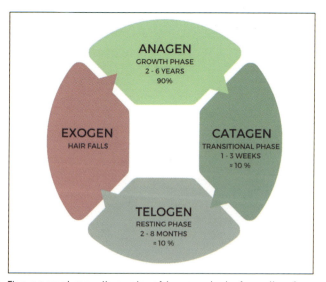

Figure 4.4. The normal growth cycle of human hair, from the Anagen phase, through the Catagen and Telogen phases, to the Exogen phase.

A hair forms in the follicle and continues to grow for two to six years until it reaches the Catagen and Telogen phases and finally falls out, and then another hair starts to grow from this follicle for another two to six years. Usually, a healthy follicle can produce 20 hairs successively before it dies. Therefore, humans can have their head of hair easily until the age of

60 to 100 years.

There are different rates of hair growth on different sections of the head; for example, the hair growth rate on the vertex, or crown, of the head is 6.2 in (16 cm) per year, whereas in the temporal area, the rate of growth is 5.5 in (14 cm) per year (Robbins, 2002, p. 9). Two important studies have compared the hair growth of Caucasians with that of Africans or African Americans. Summaries of the findings of these two studies are presented in the next sections.

## Comparison of Hair Growth Between Africans & Caucasians

**The Loussouarn study.** The Loussouarn (2001) study was one of the first scholarly attempts to compare the hair growth of Africans with that of Caucasians. This study compared the growth rates of African individuals from the African continent with that of Caucasian individuals (p. 294). Loussouarn found significant differences in the growth rates of Caucasian and African hair: African hair grew at a much slower rate than Caucasian hair (p. 297).

This study also reported that hair density in the vertex and occipital areas of African individuals was 190 ± 40 hairs per $cm^2$, whereas the hair density in the vertex and occipital areas of Caucasian individuals was 227 ± 55 hairs per $cm^2$ (Loussouarn, 2001, p. 296). According to this study, the growth rate for African individuals was 0.77 cm/month (0.30 in/month), whereas the growth rate for Caucasian individuals was 1.18 cm/month (0.47 in/month). Thus, African hair was observed to grow 35% slower than the Caucasian hair. This scientific finding corroborated the long-held complaints of African consumers regarding slower hair growth. This study also showed that the actual growth rate of hair in the Caucasian population was around 5.64 in per year, which is very close to the general perception that the growth rate is 6 in per year.

This study also reported the percentage of hairs in the Telogen phase of the two races, respectively. This Telogen percentage was reported for occipital, vertex, and temporal regions of both women and men.

In occipital regions, African women and men had a Telogen phase of 19 ± 9% versus 11 ± 7% in Caucasian women and men (Loussouarn, 2001, p. 296). In the vertex area, African women and men had a Telogen phase of 17 ± 9% versus 16 ± 13% in Caucasian men and women. When the results for the Telogen phase were pooled for both areas of the scalp, African women and men had a Telogen phase of 18 ± 9% versus 14 ± 11% in Caucasian men and women. Thus, African men and women had a significantly higher percentage of hairs in the Telogen phase.

In the temporal area, a Telogen phase of 20 ± 10% was observed for both African women and men. When analyzed by sex, African women showed a temporal Telogen phase of 16 ± 7%, while African men had a temporal Telogen phase of 25 ± 10%.

For men only, Caucasian men had a Telogen phase of 25 ± 13%, whereas African men had a Telogen phase of 20 ± 9%. Women in both races seemed to be less affected with androgenetic alopecia (AGA) than men (Loussouarn, 2001, p. 297).

**The Lewallen et al. study.** Another study was conducted by Lewallen et al. in 2015, in which the researchers compared hair growth, Anagen and Telogen phases, and the blood flow in the scalp of African-Americans and Caucasians in the United States of America (Lewallen et al., 2015, p. 216). The growth rate of hair in Caucasian women was 0.330 mm/per day, as compared to 0.259 mm/per day for African-American women (p. 219). The hair growth of African-American women was, thus, 21.52% slower than that of Caucasian women. In the Loussouarn (2001) study, the growth rate of hair of Africans from Africa was found to be 35% slower than that of Caucasians, which denoted an even larger gap.

The Lewallen et al. (2015) study also reported that Caucasian women had, on average, 37 more hairs in a 1.0 $cm^2$ area of the scalp than African-American women (p. 219). The blood flow in the scalp of Caucasian women was significantly higher than in African-American women (p. 220), which may be responsible for the higher hair growth rate among Caucasian women. Upon combing, the average number of broken fibers was 146.6 for African-American women and 13.13 for Caucasian women (p. 219). Surprisingly, this study found no difference in the number of hairs in the Anagen and Telogen phases between the two groups.

In conclusion, the rate of hair growth in African men and women is slower than in Caucasians. The hair of African men and women stays in the Telogen phase for a longer period of time as compared with the hair of Caucasian individuals. African men and women also have a much higher percentage of their hair in the Telogen phase in the temporal and occipital region than Caucasian men and women. The rate of hair growth is 35% slower in African men and women, when compared to Caucasian men and women, as reported in the Loussouarn (2001) study, and 21.52% slower, according to Lewallen et al. (2015). A dire need is recognized to mitigate this slow hair growth and the high percentage of hair in the Telogen phase in African-descent men and women. In the following sections, recommendations will be presented to alleviate this slow growth and loss of hair, especially in the vertex, occipital, and temporal regions of African-descent individuals.

If the human scalp is continuously stimulated with proper nutrients and appropriate hair products are applied daily, the hair can continue to grow for a long time during the human life span. It may be possible to increase the Anagen phase and decrease the Telogen phase in African-descent men and women by using pro-growth ingredients that slow down hair loss. Before one embarks on increasing the Anagen phase in men and women, it is pertinent to understand the causes of hair loss.

## Causes of Hair Loss

Hair loss affects approximately 50% of men and women up to age 50 and beyond (Rogers & Avram, 2008, p. 547). It is necessary to understand the causes of hair loss in order to alleviate it or to increase the growth rate of hair. The following sections describe the various causes of hair loss.

### Androgenetic or Androgenic Alopecia (AGA)

An androgen is either a natural or a synthetic steroid. The major androgens for the development of males are testosterone, dihydrotestosterone, and androstenedione. Androgens increase in both boys and girls during puberty. Although androgens are considered to be male sex hormones, they exist in females as well, but to a lesser degree. Androgens are precursors of estrogens in both men and women. The loss of hair due to androgen activity is called androgenic or androgenetic alopecia (AGA). The particular androgen responsible for hair loss is called dihydrotestosterone (DHT).

AGA is associated with aging. As women age and reach their menopausal stage, estrogen production decreases, and the enzyme 5-α-reductase converts testosterone to DHT. The accumulation of DHT leads to hair loss. There are two types of 5-α-reductase, namely, Type 1 and Type 2.

**Testosterone + 5-α-reductase → DHT → hair thinning & shedding**

In one estimate, about 10% of the testosterone in the body irreversibly converts to DHT (Dhariwala & Ravikumar, 2019, p. 966). DHT, a waxy material, causes chronic inflammation and fibrosis of the hair bulb. It continues to squeeze the hair bulb, thereby miniaturizing it and, thus, reducing the number of hair follicles, which results in hair loss (**Figure 4.5**).

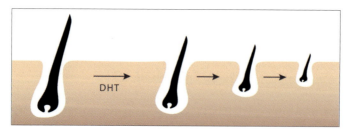

Figure 4.5. The miniaturization of the hair bulb due to the influence and action of dihydrotestosterone (DHT).

Hair loss in men is due to the change of testosterone to DHT but it is confined to the temporal-frontal occipital areas. Whereas in women, hair loss and thinning occurs primarily in the central area of the scalp, called the vertex. The Savin scale is used to categorize hair balding (i.e., AGA) in women, as shown in **Figure 4.6** (Savin, 1992, p. 604). This type of hair loss is gradual, increases with age, and depends on family history; it does not however depend on hair styling techniques. For African-American patients, a scale was devised that addressed the degree of hair

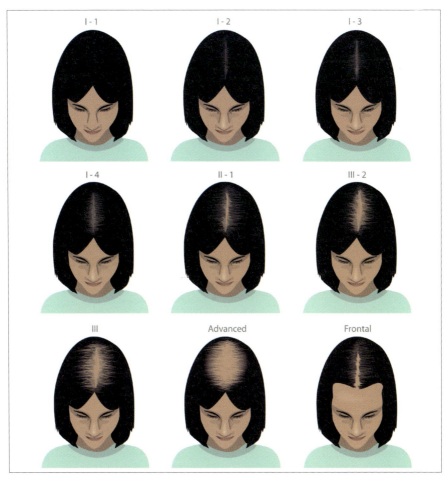

**Figure 4.6.** The Savin Scale categorizes the degree of baldness in women.

loss for individuals with curly/coily hair (Olsen et al., 2008, p. 265).

## Traction Alopecia

Traction alopecia (TA) is hair loss that occurs around the hair line and the temple area. For African-American women this usually occurs when the hair is pulled back with great tension or force for a long period of time (Khumalo & Ngwanya, 2006, p. 433). Thus, TA occurs when tensile forces are applied to pull the hair when consumers wear protective styles such as hair braiding, hair weaves, and locks (McMichael, 2003, p. 635). Excessive hair brushing, cornrowing, and the use of rollers and

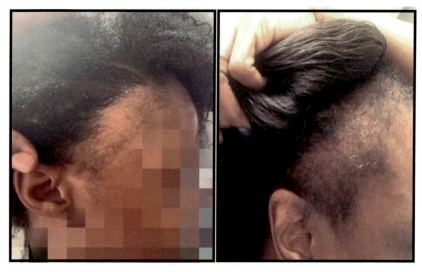

**Figure 4.7.** Traction alopecia (TA) in the temporal region of a young African-American woman in her 20s on the left and a middle-aged woman in her late 30s on the right. Courtesy of Avlon® Research Center.

hair extensions glued or clipped in place can also be responsible for TA (Whiting, 1999, p. 39). Reversible or irreversible hair loss can also result from constant manipulation of the hair line, or when the hair is pulled back into a ponytail and high viscosity gels are applied that may contain scalp-damaging ingredients such as alcohols, which can dry the scalp excessively and cause TA (Ozcelik, 2005, p. 325). Some individuals also pull their hair constantly because of a nervous condition, which results in TA. It is rather common to see African-American women experiencing significant hair loss in the temporal region, even at a young age. Two examples of TA are shown in **Figure 4.7**: the image of the left displays an African-American woman in her 20s, and the image of the right displays an African-American women in her late 30s. Both women showed significant hair loss in the temporal region, which was attributed to wearing braids in which the patients' hair was pulled back with great tensile force and kept in the braided form for a few months. This type of TA is also known as *traumatic* alopecia and can be reversed in the early stages with the use of Minoxidil solution (Khumalo & Ngwanya, 2006, p. 433).

## Alopecia Areata

Alopecia areata is a condition in which the immune system attacks the hair follicles. It manifests itself as small, round, quarter-size patches, where the hair fibers have fallen out. In some cases hair loss is more extensive. While no cure for alopecia areata currently exists, several medical treatments such as baricitinib (Olumiant®) are available to help hair grow back more quickly. A mixture of natural ingredients such as flavonoids (anthocyanidins) extracted from forbidden black rice, saw palmetto extract, beta-sitosterol, and copper tripeptide all aid in growing hair back (Avlon Research Center, 2023).

### Central Centrifugal Cicatricial Alopecia

The most common form of scarring alopecia is Central Centrifugal Cicatricial Alopecia (CCCA), which can result in permanent hair loss from the scalp. Middle-aged, African-descent women are most affected by CCCA, however this type of hair loss is seen in men and people of all races. More research needs to be conducted to determine the exact cause of CCCA. A genetic component has been suggested, with a link to mutations of the gene PADI3, which encodes peptidyl arginine deiminase, type III (PADI3), an enzyme that modifies proteins that are essential to formation of the hair-shaft. It is possible that certain hair care practices (hot combing, relaxers, tight waves, etc.) can contribute to CCCA but no conclusive link has been established. Bacterial and fungal infections, auto-immune disease, genetics, and even type 2 diabetes mellitus have been proposed as causes of CCCA. It is important to see a dermatologist for proper diagnosis and establishment of an effective treatment plan. CCCA can be reversed only if the hair follicle has not scarred. Treatment plans include the use of corticosteroids, calcineurin inhibitors, or certain antibiotics to reduce inflammation, coupled with Minoxidil to grow back hair.

### Chemically Induced Alopecia

The frequent use of chemical treatments such as permanent waves, permanent hair colors, hair lighteners, and hair relaxers, can affect the scalp negatively if applied incorrectly. Most of these treatments can alter the pH, moisture, and TEWL of the scalp. They can also induce low levels of erythema to the scalp. If used incorrectly, they may cause irritation of the scalp. A review of the literature produced several reports of cosmetic alopecia where chemicals such as hair lighteners and hair relaxers were improperly used. For example, Nicholson, Harland, Bull, Mortimer, and Cook (1993) reported that hair lighteners have high concentrations of hydrogen peroxide and powder persulfates at a high pH and an application time of approximately 45–60 minutes on the hair and off the scalp. The contact of hydrogen peroxide and bleaching powder with the scalp for a few minutes during the rinsing period of the hair lightener can cause minor oxidation of the scalp surface. Similarly, hair relaxers containing sodium hydroxide or guanidine hydroxide may irritate the scalp, reduce scalp moisture, and increase TEWL and erythema, if applied incorrectly. The exposure of the scalp to relaxer cream is normally 7 to 10 minutes, during which scalp moisture may decrease and scalp TEWL may increase. Using an after-relaxer low pH shampoo and conditioner can normalize the moisture and TEWL of the scalp. According to the manufacturers, a mixture of petrolatum and mineral oil is applied to the scalp before applying the relaxer to hair. This application of petrolatum helps in protecting the scalp from negative side effects of the relaxer cream. Petrolatum application also helps prevent scalp irritation and scarring alopecia of the vertex (Nicholson et al., 1993, p. 537).

It is, therefore, prudent to use chemical treatments with caution and less frequency. It is advisable to visit a trained hairstylist who is an expert in chemical application and aftercare. In order to avoid chemical alopecia, one should have a professional apply the chemicals and base (i.e. cover) the entire scalp in petrolatum prior to chemical application; use chemicals that are milder on the scalp; and make sure to bring the pH, moisture, and TEWL values of the hair and scalp back to their natural level with the use of low-pH-normalizing shampoos and conditioners.

## Dandruff and Seborrheic Dermatitis

Dandruff and seborrheic dermatitis can also cause hair loss in women. Dandruff is a condition that causes the skin cells on the scalp to flake. The exact cause of dandruff is still unclear but generally dandruff has

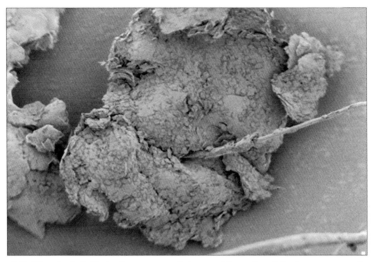

**Figure 4.8.** The hair follicle becomes thin and barely able to emerge from the interior of the scalp (x1550). Photo courtesy of Avlon® Research Center.

been associated with the prescence of a fungus of the *Malassezia species* on the scalp. The *Malassezia* fungus is lipophillic and feeds on oil and sebum on the scalp. When the cells of the scalp turn over at a much faster rate, they form a layer on the scalp. Underneath this layer, moisture and sebum collect, providing a perfect environment for further growth of fungus and bacteria on the scalp, which may lead to biofilm formation. This fungus makes the scalp itchy, and the excessive turnover of cells starts to peel away from the scalp and fall onto the shoulders, making an unappealing sight. In African-descent consumers, dandruff is prevalent from the age of 15 to 50 years, and in one estimate, half of the African-descent population suffers from dandruff along with itchy scalp (Cardin, 1998, p. 193). The large flakes can become obstructive to hair growth, as shown in **Figure 4.8**.

Seborrheic dermatitis (SD), widely considered as an exacerbated form of dandruf, affects not only the scalp but the face and other parts of the body too. Additionally, SD is accompanied by inflammation and erythema of the skin. The scalp is coated with a very heavy, sticky, and greasy film that inflames the surface (Elewski, 2005, p. 190), and interferes with the growth of hair (Levin & Behrman, 1946, p. 90). The sticky white film is shown in **Figure 4.9(a)**. The inflammation resulting from scratching the itchy scalp is shown in **Figure 4.9(b)**. Individuals suffering from dandruff,

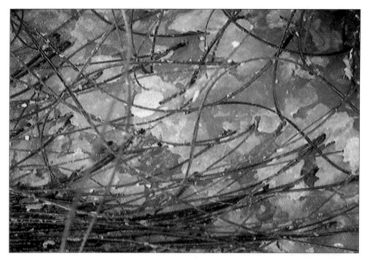

**Figure 4.9(a).** Image of a scalp containing a sticky film of dandruff. The dandruff film was very hard to remove even with the use of dandruff shampoos. Scalp image taken using a handheld contact microscope. Photo courtesy of Avlon® Research Center.

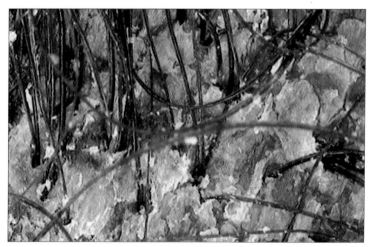

**Figure 4.9(b).** Image of a scalp containing a sticky film of dandruff and scarring. Due to biofilm formation on the scalp, the patient scratched the scalp with her nails, producing red, irritated areas; here, visible as dark spots around two hair cavities. With frequent scratching, these two areas can become scarred and lead to the loss of hair growth. Scalp image taken using a handheld contact microscope. Photo courtesy of Avlon® Research Center.

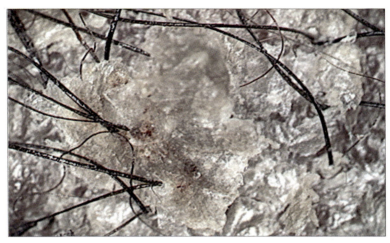

Figure 4.10. Image of a scalp containing dandruff flakes, red spots and scars from itching. The excessive scratching of the scalp produced scars that decreased the hair density. The craters on the scalp show that a significant number of follicles have died. Photo courtesy of Avlon® Research Center.

or seborrheic dermatitis, experience frequent itching of the scalp that leads to frequent scratching with the fingernails. The scars produced by scratching are responsible for the hair loss, shown in **Figure 4.10**.

## Menopause

Another cause of hair loss in women is menopause. Estrogen production decreases in women when they reach the age of menopause and hair growth slows down significantly, resulting in hair loss.

## Diet Deficiencies or Overload

Diet deficiencies also affect the growth of hair. If the nutrient supply to hair follicles in the food intake is either deficient or overloaded, hair loss can occur. It is widely known that deficiency of one or more nutrients such as iron, zinc, niacin (Vitamin B3), fatty acids, selenium, Vitamin D, Vitamin A, folic acid, biotin, and L-lysine may be the cause of hair loss (Guo & Katta, 2017, p. 2). The overload of certain nutrients such as iron can also cause hair loss. It is, therefore, recommended that a balanced diet, based on proteins, complex carbohydrates, iron, vitamins, and minerals, be consumed because it may optimize the growth of hair.

Studies conducted over the last decade have shown that phytosterols such as beta-sitosterol can help the growth of hair and significantly alleviate shedding and thinning (Prager, Bicket, French, & Marcovici, 2002, p. 17). Beta-sitosterol is generally present in natural oils such as liposterolic extract of *Serenoa repens* (saw palmetto berries), pumpkin seed oil, almond oil, watermelon seed oil, rice bran oil, soybean oil, peanut oil, and others. Beta-sitosterol can now be found as a supplement in the marketplace; it is also added to foods such as juices and yogurts, among others.

### Other Health Issues

Conditions such as high fever, hormonal imbalance, medications, stress, and chemotherapy can result in hair loss. A proper analysis of the cause of hair loss is required in order to mitigate it.

## Treating Hair Loss & Hair Loss Remedies

As mentioned before, the cause of hair loss among African-descent women in the United States and elsewhere occurs mainly due to androgenetic alopecia, followed by traction alopecia (from braids and weaves), alopecia areata, central centrifugal cicatricial alopecia, dandruff/seborrheic dermatitis, and chemically induced alopecia due to excessive use of chemically reactive products such as hair colors, hair lighteners, and hair straighteners. This hair loss can be managed if a mitigation plan is followed early in life. If patients suffering from hair loss do not seek help in the early years of their lives, the hair loss becomes irreversible. Various remedies available against hair loss are discussed in the next section.

Remedies for hair loss can be based on drugs, botanical ingredients, and surgical options. Effective drugs approved by FDA include Minoxidil, Finasteride, Dutasteride, and a combination of Minoxidil and Tretinoin. Successful botanical ingredients to treat hair loss are saw palmetto extract, beta-sitosterol, flavonoids such as anthocyanidins from forbidden black rice, Copper Tripeptides, but they are not approved by FDA. Surgical options are hair transplants, which are very expensive and painful.

## Medical Treatments

**Minoxidil.** The most common drug used for the alleviation of hair loss is Minoxidil. Interestingly, Minoxidil was originally used in the late 1970s as an oral drug for treating high blood pressure. Minoxidil is *piperidinopyrimidine derivative* with the specific chemical structure of 2,6-diamino-4-piperidinopyrimidine 1-oxide, shown in **Figure 4.11**.

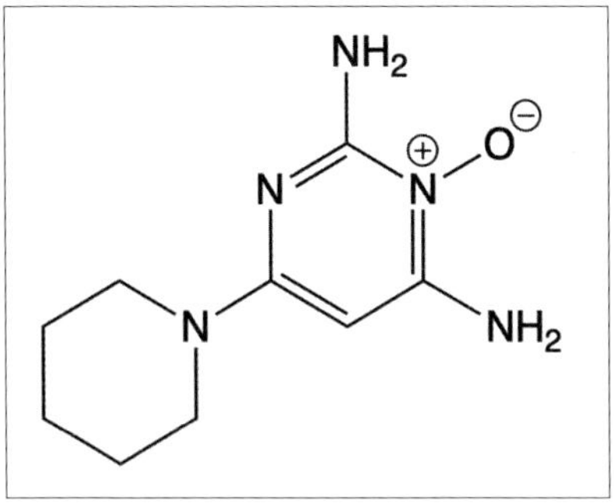

Figure 4.11. Structure of Minoxidil, which consists of 2,6-diamino-4-piperidinopyrimidine 1-oxide.

Minoxidil serves as a vasodilator to open potassium channels. In one study of 100 patients, it produced unwanted hair growth in 24% of the patients (Jacomb & Brunnberg, 1976, S580). In another study with 15 patients, hypertrichosis (excessive hair growth) was observed in all patients (Dargie, Dollery, & Daniel, 1977, p. 518). Hypertrichosis was also noted in five out of six pediatric patients who were treated with Minoxidil (Pennisi et al., 1977, p. 817). Even in women, who had received lower doses than men, hypertrichosis was observed (Jacobs & Buttigieg, 1981, p. 477).

Based on these findings, several studies were conducted using Minoxidil as a topical treatment for alopecia areata (AA). Alopecia areata is a common autoimmune skin disease causing hair loss on the scalp, face, and sometimes other parts of the body. In 1984, five patients with androgenetic alopecia and 10 patients with alopecia areata were randomly treated with 1% or 5% topical Minoxidil or a placebo. The study results showed that 60% of the androgenetic alopecia patients treated with 5% Minoxidil regrew their hair. The cultures of human epidermal cells that were treated with Minoxidil survived longer than control cultures, and it was also found that thinning of the keratinocytes (senescence) slowed down and the cells stayed in the germinative pool for longer periods (Baden & Kubilus, 1983, p. 560). It was also found that Minoxidil increased the dermal papilla cells of human hair follicles, thereby, stimulating growth, prolonging the Anagen phase, and elongating hair fibers (Han et al., 2004, p. 97). Another study claimed that the Anagen:Telogen ratio increased along with the hair fiber diameter when 2.0% and 3.0% Minoxidil solution was used for a year (Abell, 1988, p. 193). In the case of traction alopecia, a study with two subjects showed significant hair growth with 2.0% topical Minoxidil (Khumalo & Ngwanya, 2006, p. 433). Currently, androgenetic alopecia is also treated with 2.5 mg per day oral Minoxidil for women. Men would require a slightly higher dose of 5 mg.

**Side effects of Minoxidil.** One of the side effects of Minoxidil is hypertrichosis, which means the growth of hair on unwanted areas such as on a woman's face. Other side effects could be allergic contact dermatitis, scalp irritation, and seborrheic dermatitis. Contact dermatitis may be caused by propylene glycol, present in the Minoxidil solution (Friedman, Friedman, Cohen, & Washenik, 2002, p. 309). Similarly, seborrheic dermatitis may be caused by the presence of ethanol in the Minoxidil solution, where the ethanol most likely dries out African-descent hair significantly. Minoxidil is not recommended when a woman is pregnant or breastfeeding. One report indicated that a pregnant woman could give birth to a child with hypertrichosis (Veyrec et al., 1995, p. 474).

**Combination of Minoxidil and Tretinoin.** According to Ferry, Forbes, James, Vanderlugt, and Szpunar (1990, p. 446), when Tretinoin Cream (0.05% active) was used 1x a day in conjunction with 2.0% Minoxidil

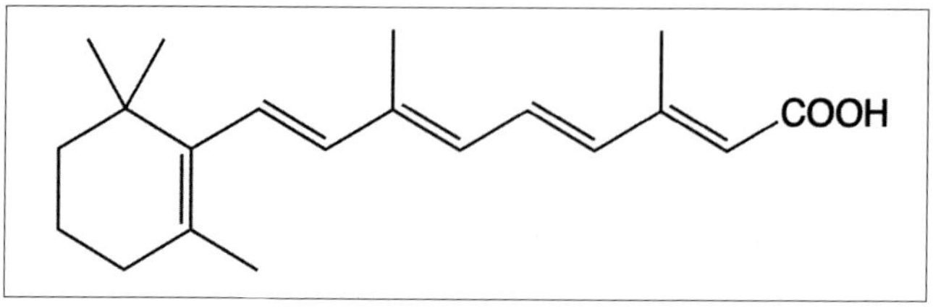

Figure 4.12. Structure of Tretinoin (commonly known as retinoic acid).

2x a day, the absorption of Minoxidil increased 3 fold versus 1.3 fold with a vehicle carrying Minoxidil. When a 5% solution of Minoxidil was used along with 0.01% Tretinoin, the frequency of daily application was reduced to 1x a day with the same effect as the 2x a day use of Minoxidil (Shin et al., 2007, p. 290).

Tretinoin (see **Figure 4.12** for structure) is a naturally occuring derivative of Vitamin A and although its exact mechanism of hair growth is unknown, it was reported that retinoic acid increases the growth factors involved in the initiation, differentiation, and inhibition of hair follicle growth (Bergfeld, 1998, p. S87).

One side effect of the combination of Minoxidil and Tretinoin was an increase in TEWL, which can eventually lead to dry skin.

**Finasteride.** Another drug that is effective against hair loss, but for men only, is Finasteride (see **Figure 4.13** for structure). The dosage is 1 mg per day. This drug was approved by the FDA in 1997. It is prescribed as an oral remedy for hair loss.

Drake et al. (1999, p. 551) tested 0.01 mg to 5.0 mg of Finasteride per day on 245 participants. Two types of 5-α reductase exist, identified as Type 1 and Type 2, where Type 1 is simply 5-α reductase, and Type 2 is called isoenzyme of 5-a α reductase. The two types of 5-α reductase convert testosterone to DHT. The scalp contains Type 1, 5-α reductase,

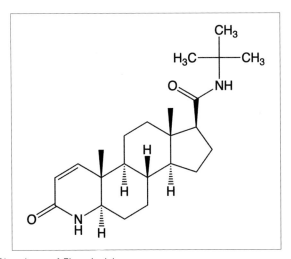

Figure 4.13. Structure of Finasteride.

whereas Type 2, 5-α reductase is present in the connective sheaths and dermal papillae of hair follicles. Finasteride inhibits Type 2, 5-α reductase. It is noted that male-pattern baldness does not take place in men who are genetically deficient in Type 2, 5-α reductase. The Drake et al. study indicated that 0.2 mg per day of Finasteride decreased scalp DHT levels by 60% to 70% over a 6-week period. Based on this data, a group of investigators evaluated various doses between 0.2 mg and 1.0 mg per day (Roberts et al., 1999, p. 562). They concluded that, for male-pattern baldness, 1.0 mg was the optimal daily dose.

**Side effects of Finasteride.** Rogers & Avram (2008) reported:
- Because of the risk of feminizing a male fetus, Finasteride should not be taken by women of childbearing age.
- Sexual side effects for men are decreased libido, erectile dysfunction, and ejaculation disorder.
- Unusual side effects were exfoliative dermatitis, perioral numbness, and swollen glands.

All of these side effects stopped when drug intake was discontinued (Rogers & Avram (2008) pp. 554-556).

**Dutasteride.** The Dutasteride molecule is similar to Finasteride. The chemical structure of Dutasteride is shown in **Figure 4.14**.

As mentioned earlier, Finasteride inhibits Type 2, 5-α reductase, whereas 5.0 mg per day Dutasteride inhibits both Type 1, and Type 2, 5-α reductase. Therefore, Dutasteride is three times more effective in inhibiting Type 2, 5-α reductase than Finasteride, and 100 times more effective in inhibiting Type 1, 5-α reductase. A study was conducted with 399 patients suffering from prostate enlargement in 33 medical centers in the USA (Clark et al., 2004). The investigation also determined an optimum dose of Dutasteride. Upon the final results, it was concluded that Dutasteride inhibited both types of 5-α reductase with almost complete suppression of DHT (p. 2183).

Some of the side effects of Dutasteride were altered libido, headaches, and impotence. These side effects were similar to those of Finasteride in general (Clark et al., 2004, p. 2183).

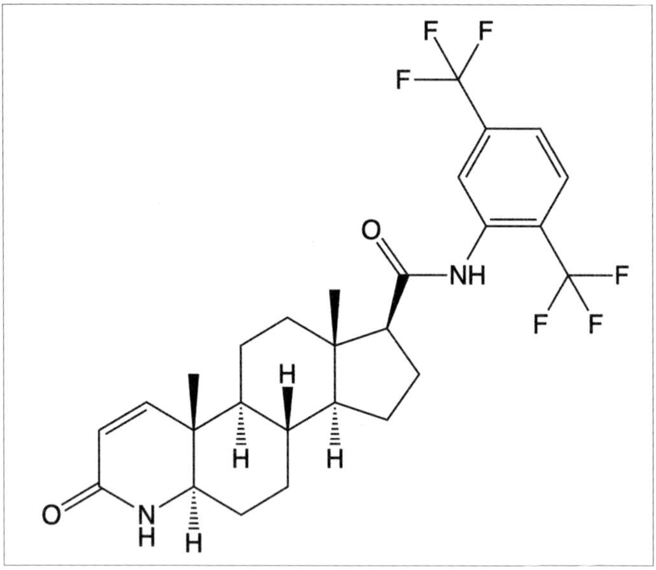

Figure 4.14. Structure of Dutasteride.

## Alternative Botanical Treatments (Non-FDA Approved)

**Saw palmetto extract (85%–95%).** One of the early studies on botanical treatments of hair loss was published by Prager et al., in 2002. The researchers used beta-sitosterol and liposterolic extract of *Serenoa repens* (LSESr) to control AGA in men and women (p. 8). The study was based on a mixture of 50 mg of beta-sitosterol and 200 mg of liposterolic extract of *Serenoa repens* (LSESr–85%-95% extract) as active ingredients and placed in a capsule. The daily dose was two capsules. It was tested on a total of 19 patients, where nine patients received a placebo and 10 patients received the actual drug. The study was conducted for 18 to 24.7 weeks, and 60% of the patients reported improvement in their hair growth, as compared to the baseline (p. 16).

According to one study, *Serenoa repens* was a potent inhibitor of the activity of both Type 1, and Type 2, 5-α reductase isoenzymes, which was similar to the effect of Dutasteride (Habib, Ross, Ho, Lyons, & Chapman, 2005, p. 192). However, some studies indicated that *Serenoa repens* was not effective against benign prostatic hyperplasia (Bent et al., 2006, p. 557; MacDonald, Tacklind, Rutks, & Wilt, 2012, p. 1756). These finding cast a shadow on the effectiveness of saw palmetto against androgenetic alopecia, considering that the chemistry underlying the reaction in both benign prostatic hyperplasia and androgenetic alopecia is the same.

**Beta-sitosterol.** Natural extracts or oils that are rich in beta-sitosterol are effective against hair loss 60% to 70% of the time. Oils such as pumpkinseed oil and saw palmetto extract are reasonable choices. If these oils are mixed with beta-sitosterol, the shedding and thinning of hair stops significantly (Avlon® study, 2010, unpublished).

Over the last decade, beta-sitosterol has been available as a stand-alone ingredient at active concentrations of 50% to 75%. Thus, formulating chemists are able to combine beta-sitosterol with natural oils. They can also formulate creams and lotions for daily use by adding phytosterols with an activity of 25 to 50 mg per gram.

**Biotin.** The literature indicates that administering biotin orally (10-30 mg daily) resolved any nail disorders in horses (Comben et al., 1984, p. 642). However, when biotin was studied in connection with human hair growth, it did not result in any improvement to the growth of hair (Limat et al., 1996, p. 31). Thus, the popular belief that biotin helps to grow hair is not supported by scientific studies.

**Copper.** One in-vitro study found that the copper-tripeptide complex (L-alanyl-L-histidyl-L-lysine-$Cu^2$) promoted hair growth in laboratory experiments (Pyo et al., 2007, p. 834). The copper complex stimulated the proliferation of dermal papilla cells (DPC), which are important in the growth of hair follicles. This stimulation was responsible for the elongation of human hair follicles. The complex decreased the number of apoptotic dermal papilla cells, but the decrease was not statistically significant.

In an animal study, C3H mice were injected with the peptide-copper complex intradermally, while the controls were injected with a saline solution. The results showed that the Telogen phase was reduced and the Anagen phase increased with the peptide-copper complex injection (Trachy, Fors, Pickart, & Uno, 1991, p. 469).

**Green Tea.** Oxidative stresses have been linked to hair loss (Guo &

Katta, 2017, p. 6). The Latin name or the name featured in the International Nomenclature of Cosmetic Ingredients (INCI) for Green Tea is *camellia sinensis*. Green Tea is processed from unfermented tea leaves and found to have high concentrations of polyphenols as antioxidants (Draelos, 2010, p. 68). Most antioxidants are anti-inflammatory as well. Eigallocatechin-3-gallate (EGCG) is a potent polyphenol and found abundantly in white, caffeine-free, Green Tea powder. The EGCG in Green Tea is not stable for very long in aqueous solution (Hsu, 2005, p. 1056); therefore, the powder form of Green Tea should be added to oral formulations. Green Tea alone will not be able to grow hair, but when combined with active hair growth ingredients it may improve growth.

**Aloe vera gel.** Aloe vera juice is widely used in skin care and cosmetic ingredients as an anti-inflammatory substance. It is obtained by squeezing aloe vera leaves to obtain a colorless liquid gel, which contains 99.5% water and a mixture of mucopolysaccharides, amino acids, hydroxy quinone glycosides, and minerals (Draelos, 2010, p. 72). Many studies have been conducted on the anti-inflammatory effect of aloe vera gel on the human skin. Aloe vera gel has scientifically demonstrated its anti-

Table 4.2 *Advantages and Disadvantages of Alternative Botanical Treatments for Hair Loss*

| Advantages |
|---|
| Holistic solution addressing thinning and shedding concerns |
| Can be administered orally |
| Can be administered as active ingredients in shampoos, conditioners, topical lotions, creams, or oils |
| Not drying to the hair and scalp because they do not contain alcohol or propylene glycol |
| Can promote a healthy scalp enviroment for hair growth and restoration |

| Disadvantages |
|---|
| Cannot make hair growth claims due to FDA guidelines and regulations |

inflammatory activity and can be used in folk medicine for the treatment of inflammations of the skin (Vazquez et al., 1996, p. 74). It is the experience of this author that 20% of aloe vera gel in water significantly reduces redness and irritation of the scalp, caused by irritants such as alkaline hair bleaches and relaxers.

**Iron.** Iron deficiency (ID) may result in hair loss (Guo & Katta, 2017, p. 1). First of all, the patient must be tested for iron deficiency before taking iron supplements because taking more iron than your body needs can cause serious medical problems. Iron deficiency is more prevalent in African Americans. Co-consumption of Vitamin C enhances iron absorption, while phytate found in cereals inhibits iron absorption. As mentioned previously, hair follicle matrix cells divide very rapidly and could be more sensitive to iron deficiency, which could result in hair loss (Trost et al., 2006, p. 824). In the Rushton, Norris, Dover, and Busuttil (2002) study, patients suffering from iron and lysine imbalance were given Florisene® iron supplement, which reduced hair shedding by 61% at $p < .001$ (p. 22).

**Zinc.** Almost 300 enzymes in the body require zinc to contribute to human growth, development, wound healing, immune function, and collagen synthesis. The body cannot synthesize zinc; therefore, it is considered an essential nutrient and must be taken orally. Certain medicines such as diuretics may lower zinc levels (Goldberg & Lenzy, 2010, p. 413). Persons diagnosed with low serum zinc levels may suffer from alopecia areata; thus, zinc supplements could help alleviate hair loss (Goldberg & Lenzy, 2010, p. 413; Park at al., 2009, p. 142).

**Niacin (Vitamin $B_3$).** Alopecia is one of the results of Niacin deficiency (Guo & Katta, 2017, p. 3). However, Niacin is now widely used in skin care products to condition the skin and also help the adsorption of cosmetically active ingredients in topical scalp treatments.

**Fatty acids.** In many cases, changes in skin and hair signal a deficiency in vitamins and other essential nutrients. For example, deficiency of polyunsaturated essential fatty acids such omega 3 (alpha-linolenic acid) and omega 6 (linoleic acid) can result in hair loss from the scalp and eyebrows, along with lightening of the hair (Goldberg & Lenzy, 2010, p. 413).

**Selenium.** Evidence regarding hair loss due to selenium deficiency is almost nonexistent; only one study showed that a Japanese child suffered sparse, short, thin, light-colored hair growth due to selenium deficiency (Kenekura et al., 2005, p. 346). His skin lesions responded to supplemental treatment with sodium selenite ($Na_2SeO_3$). His skin symptoms were similar to symptoms of zinc deficiency.

As a nutrient, selenium exists in the human body in minute quantities. In one study, nine patients were tested for a large presence of selenium from taking liquid supplements. These large amounts of selenium in the human body resulted in adverse reactions, where one of the symptoms was hair loss in four out of nine patients (Aldosary, Sutter, Schwartz, & Morgan, 2012, p. 59). It is, therefore, not advisable to take selenium in supplements, unless the selenium deficiency is well-documented through clinical testing.

**Vitamin D**. Low levels of Vitamin D, like iron deficiency, are responsible for hair loss (Rasheed et al., 2013, p. 105). It is important to monitor Vitamin D levels through regular blood analysis once every 6 months to 1 year because an optimal level of Vitamin D is necessary to delay hair loss.

**Vitamin A**. The role of Vitamin A in combination with Minoxidil has been discussed previously in this chapter. An excess of Vitamin A triggers hair loss (Everts, 2012, p. 222).

**Vitamin E**. Very little information is available about Vitamin E intake and its relationship with hair loss. Beoy, Eoei, and Hay (2010, p. 91) observed that patients suffering from alopecia exhibited lower levels of antioxidants in their scalp area and also a higher lipid peroxidation index. The patients were given 100 mg of mixed tocotrienols daily for 8 months. The results showed a 34.5% increase in the number of hairs when compared with placebo takers.

**Folic acid.** According to Durusoy et al. (2009, p. 790), 91 patients with diffuse hair loss and 74 healthy individuals were studied, and the levels of their folate, zinc, and Vitamin $B_{12}$ were compared. The authors did not find any correlation between hair loss and deficiencies in folates, zinc, and vitamin $B_{12}$.

**Amino acids and proteins.** The amino acid L-lysine possibly plays a role in iron and zinc uptake. When L-lysine was added to iron supplements, the ferritin concentration increased in women suffering from iron deficiency and Telogen effluvium (TE). No credible studies were found to indicate that taking amino acids or proteins will help in reducing hair loss.

In summary, patients should be tested first for any deficiency in nutrients. Then, supplements containing these nutrients could be utilized for proper hair loss treatment. Caution must be exercised because excessive intake of Vitamin A, Vitamin E, and selenium could result in hair loss (Guo & Katta, 2017, p. 8).

**Treatment of Seborrheic Dermatitis/Dandruff.** As discussed above, dandruff and seborrheic dermatitis can lead to hair loss. They can be effectively treated with over-the-counter (OTC) shampoos and conditioners. FDA guidelines require products that treat dandruff and seborrheic dermatitis to contain at least one of the following active ingredients:

- **Zinc Pyrithione.** 0.50% to 2.0% in rinse-off products for seborrheic dermatitis. Zinc pyrithione is not allowed in Europe now.
- **Selenium Sulfide.** 1.0% for rinse-off products.
- **Ketoconazole.** 1.0% to 2.0% for rinse-off products. A medicated shampoo with 2.0% ketoconazole appears to enhance hair growth if used with 2.0% Minoxidil, when compared to just 2.0% Minoxidil without the use of a medicated shampoo (Pierard-Franchimont, De Donker, Cauwenbergh, & Pierard, 1998, p. 477).

- **Salicylic Acid.** 1.8% to 3.0% for seborrheic dermatitis and psoriasis.
- **Sulfur.** 2% to 5%.
- **Coal Tar Extract.** 0.5% to 5%. However, coal tar is now known as a carcinogen; its use is, therefore, banned in Europe and many states in the USA.

The most popular ingredient for dandruff and seborrheic dermatitis is Zinc Pyrithione at 1.0% in a shampoo and/or conditioner base. The base of the shampoo must be designed differently for African-American hair and scalp: These shampoos must contain more moisturizing ingredients (McMichael, 2003, p. 639). A dandruff shampoo should be used once a week, not daily, and it should be followed by a dandruff conditioner containing 0.5% to 1.0% active Zinc Pyrithione. The shampoo should be applied to the scalp first and left on the scalp for 5–10 minutes, followed by lathering with fingers, then rinsed, and repeated. An antidandruff conditioner should be applied to hair and scalp and left on for 15–20 minutes before rinsing.

Other non-OTC, antidandruff ingredients that effectively remove dandruff from the scalp are piroctone olamine and bis-pyrithione. Neither of these ingredients is approved by the FDA, although piroctone olamine is approved in Europe and Asia.

## Surgical Hair Transplants

Hair transplants are a surgical technique where hair follicles are transferred from the back of the head to the frontal area, or to the bald spot. The place from which the hair follicles are taken is called the *donor site,* and the frontal bald area of the head is known as the *recipient site.* This technique is normally used to treat male-pattern baldness, or androgenetic alopecia, which exists in both men and women. The doner sites are usually resistant to male-pattern baldness, and grafts containing follicles are surgically harvested and transferred to the bald spot of the head. Hair loss from causes other than male-pattern baldness (e.g., illness, burns, accidents, or operations) can also be treated with hair transplantation.

Surgical techniques include the following: Hair transplantation, micro- and minitransplants, and scalp reduction.

**Hair transplantation.** The patient is instructed to keep hair long at donor and recipient sites. The patient uses an antiseptic shampoo for 3 days before the surgery. The day of the surgery, the patient is given light anesthesia, and donor and recipient sites are scrubbed with antiseptic soap. The donor transplants are removed at the lowest depth and transplanted on the recipient site of the carefully planned hairline. In order for hair growth to be successful, the placement of grafts is a very important step (Roenigk, 1998, p. 634).

**Micro- and minitransplants.** Micro- and minitransplants are often performed after a hair transplant to soften the hair line, fill in between the larger grafts, and fill in the "cornstalk" appearance (Roenigk, 1998, p. 636). In this case, the hair grafts are smaller, but the surgical procedure is the same as in the hair transplantation.

**Scalp reduction.** Scalp reduction is a technique similar to hair transplantation. It is performed on patients who have their frontal hair still intact, but the vertex is balding. Here, the scalp is surgically reduced, and the balding area is decreased or eliminated. This surgery is more intensive, and removal of the bald spot is accomplished with multiple surgeries, rather than just one operation (McCray & Roenigk, 1983, p. 207).

### Hairpieces and Wigs

To camouflage the bald spot of the scalp, hair pieces are prepared and then attached temporarily onto the scalp. The technology of preparing and attaching these hair pieces has significantly evolved to where they look quite natural and are aesthetically appealing. It is now very fashionable for women to attach pieces of human hair to their existing hair to gain length and an appealing appearance. This is accomplished by gluing extensions to the existing hair by expert hairstylists.

The attachment of hair extensions has come of age and has become a booming business. The advantage of toupees, wigs, and hair pieces is that the consumer is able to get a full head of hair immediately. The disadvantage of false hair and toupees is that they are recognizable by others as such and carry a social stigma.

Curly Hair: Structure, Properties, & Care | Chapter 4

## Definition of Terms

**Alopecia areata (AA).** Alopecia areata is a common autoimmune skin disease causing hair loss on the scalp, face, and sometimes on other parts of the body.

**Aloe Vera.** Aloe vera is a stemless green plant that can grow up to 20 or 40 in. The roots of the plant have access to the minerals of the soil. **Figure 4.15(a)** and **Figure 4.15(b)** show the plant and a cut piece of the stem, used to squeeze the juice of the plant, known as aloe vera juice or aloe vera gel. This gel is well-known for its anti-inflammatory properties.

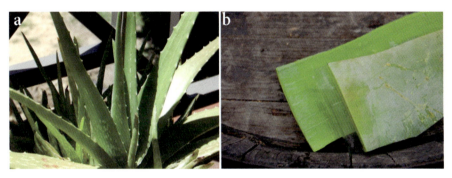

Figure 4.15. (a) Image of an aloe vera plant. (b) Image of a piece of the aloe vera plant leaf cut for squeezing out the juice (which is aloe vera gel).

Aloe vera juice contains many phytochemicals, and a plethora of scientific literature is available regarding the properties of aloe vera juice with its gellike consistency. Hundreds of cosmetic and food products include aloe vera gel as one of the ingredients in their formulations.

**Amino acids and proteins.** Amino acids are the building blocks of all proteins. The structure of an amino acid is shown in **Figure 4.16**. The acid part of one amino acid links with the amino part of the next amino group and forms a peptide bond. When multiple amino acids combine in this fashion, the resultant molecule is called a polypeptide or a protein. Many proteins are found in the human hair and scalp; they play different roles in the growth and formation of a hair strand.

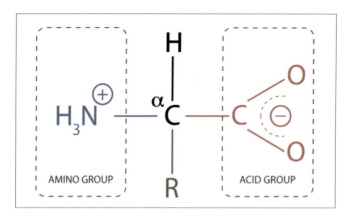

Figure 4.16. Structure of an α-amino acid.

**Anagen.** Anagen is the growth phase in the hair's growth cycle from the scalp. Starting with intense metabolic activity in the hair bulb, a hair is produced that keeps growing. The hair stays in the Anagen phase up to 90% of its existence. In **Figure 4.17**, a hair fiber is shown in the Anagen phase of its growth cycle. The root of the Anagen hair is covered by a long sheath. The patient from whom this hair was taken was 29 years old and losing his hair at the front of the head. The hair depicted was taken from the back of the patient's head.

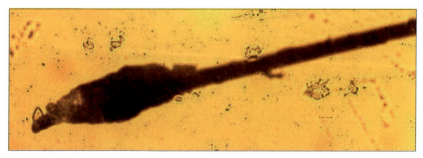

Figure 4.17. The root of the Anagen hair is covered by a long sheath, as shown on the left side of this image. Photo courtesy of Avlon® Research Center.

**Androgens.** An androgen is a natural or synthetic steroid. The major androgens for the development of males are testosterone, dihydrotestosterone, and androstenedione.

**Androgenetic or androgenic alopecia (AGA).** The loss of hair due to androgens is called androgenic or androgenetic alopecia.

**Antioxidants.** Many materials in the human body are capable of reacting with oxygen or free radicals, thereby producing undesirable by-products. Antioxidant compounds are free-radical scavengers that readily interfere, thereby stopping the oxidation processes and the unwanted production of new chemicals, which may be deleterious to the health of the body, skin, scalp, and hair. Examples of antioxidant materials are Vitamin C, Vitamin E, enzymes, glutathione, and many other such compounds.

**Arrector pili muscles.** The arrector pili muscles are small muscles attached to hair follicles. Contraction of these muscles causes the hair to stand on end (Figure 4.1).

**Basal layer.** The basal layer is the deepest layer of the five layers of the epidermis. It is composed of columnar or cuboidal basal cells. In a single layer, these cells are attached to each other and also to the top layer, called *stratum spinosum*. Some basal cells can act like stem cells that are able to divide and produce new cells. These cells are called basal keratinocyte stem cells. Basal cells also contain melanocytes (pigment producing cells), Langerhans cells (immune cells), and Markel cells (touch receptors). See **Figure 4.18**.

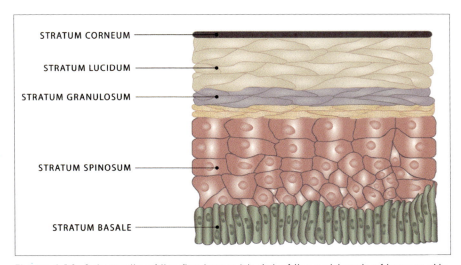

Figure 4.18. Schematic of the five layers (strata) of the epidermis of human skin.

**Beta-sitosterol.** Sterols are naturally found in plants as a combination of beta-sitosterol, campesterol, and stigmasterol. Beta-sitosterol is effective in lowering cholesterol in the human blood; thus, it helps in lowering the incidence of heart attacks. Beta-sitosterol also helps in decreasing shedding and thinning of human hair from the scalp. In the skin, beta-sitosterol helps in building the stratum corneum, consequently improving the health of the skin. It is found in various natural oils such as pumpkinseed oil.

**Biotin.** Biotin is also called Vitamin H; in some countries, it is called Vitamin 7 and Vitamin 8. It is also called a water-soluble B vitamin. Although it is used for hardening the nails of horses, it does not show any promise for improving hair growth, contrary to popular belief.

**Blood vessels.** Blood vessels are part of the circulatory system in the human body. They transport blood cells, nutrients, and oxygen to the body's tissues. They are also responsible for carrying away the waste and carbon dioxide from the tissues. There are five types of blood vessels: arteries, arterioles, capillaries, venules, veins. The functions of these five parts can be described as follows:

- Arteries carry oxygen-rich blood away from the heart;
- Arterioles are small in diameter and extend and branch out from an artery and lead to capillaries;
- Capillaries are the sites where the exchange of water and chemicals between blood and tissues takes place;
- Venules are small blood vessels in the microcirculation that allow blood to return from the capillaries to drain into large blood vessels, the veins;
- Veins carry blood from the capillaries back to the heart.

**Capillaries.** The exchange of water and chemicals (nutrients) between blood and tissues occurs in the capillaries.

**Catagen.** The Catagen phase is a transitional stage in the hair growth cycle where hair transitions from the Anagen to the Telogen (resting) phase. Only about 1% to 5% of the hair is in the Catagen phase at any given time.

**Cell differentiation.** Through cell differentiation, cells change from one cell type to another specialized type. The cells marry each other and change to complex tissues, and this differentiation continues even in adulthood as adult stem cells divide and create differentiated daughter cells during the process of tissue repair and normal cell turnover.

**Cell proliferation.** The process by which a cell grows and divides to produce two daughter cells as equal copies. Cell proliferation is responsible for the exponential increase in the number of cells.

**Chemically induced alopecia.** The use of chemicals can burn the scalp and produce scars, which may lead to permanent hair loss. Chemically induced hair loss is irreversible.

**Copper deficiency.** Deficiency in copper-tripeptides can cause hair loss that can be reversed when copper-tripeptides are taken orally.

**Dermal papilla.** Ovoid and pear-shaped, this large structure at the base of the hair follicle is located near the center of the bulb (see Figure 4.1). It plays a major role in the development of the hair follicle during the Anagen, Catagen, and Telogen phases (Robbins, 2002, p. 4).

**Epithelial tissue.** The epithelial tissue is one of the major types of tissues; it covers the surface of the human body. It has several different functions such as protection, absorption, secretion, filtration, excretion, and sensory reception. The epithelium of the skin protects underlying tissues from mechanical damage, chemical damage, and bacterial invasion.

**Exogen.** In the Exogen phase of the hair growth cycle, fibers begin to fall out, after being in the Telogen (resting) phase for a certain length of time. After the Exogen phase, the hair enters the Anagen phase again.

**Hair bulb.** The lower expanded extremity of the hair fiber; it fits like a cap over the hair papilla at the bottom portion of the follicle.

**Hair follicle matrix.** Found around the papilla and hair bulb. The hair matrix sits above the hair bulb. A hair comes into existence from a single stem cell group, called the *matrix of the hair bulb*.

**Hair transplant**. Hair follicles are surgically removed from the back of the head and transplanted to the frontal area of the head for combatting frontal hair loss. This surgical operation is called hair transplant.

**Hypertrichosis**. Hypertrichosis is the growth of hair on unwanted areas such as a woman's face, arms, neck, or chest.

**Inner root sheath (IRS)**. The inner root sheath lies between the hair bulb and the outer root sheath. It is an important structure of the lower part of the hair follicle; its role is to surround and protect the growing hair. The IRS itself is made up of three layers called Henle's layer, Huxley's layer, and the cuticle of the inner root sheath.

**Melanocytes**. Melanocytes are located just around the dermal papilla. They are pigment-producing cells; thus, the name melanocytes.

**Menopause**. Menopause is the time in a woman's life when her menstrual periods stop permanently, and she is no longer able to conceive children. On average, this occurs around the age of 49 to 52 years. The medical confirmation of menopause is the absence of menstrual bleeding for one year. The production of hormones by the ovaries decreases significantly with menopause.

**Moisture measurement of the scalp.** The moisture or hydration of the scalp is assessed by measuring the conducting properties of the very upper layers of the scalp, when subjected to alternating voltage. A probe with eight-contact pins is useful for measuring between hairs, on the scalp, or other rough and uneven surfaces. The probe has a spring-loaded action, which initiates a measurement when the probe is pressed against the scalp and the output is presented in units of micro-Siemens ($\mu$S). Six readings are taken for each subject: three readings from each side of the head and the average is calculated.

**Outer root sheath (ORS).** The outer root sheath encloses the inner root sheath and the hair shaft. The ORS continues upward to the basal layer of the epidermis. Its role is to protect the hair bulb, hair shaft, and inner root sheath.

**Sebaceous glands.** The sebaceous glands are exocrine glands that open into a hair follicle and secrete an oily or waxy matter, called *sebum*, which lubricates and waterproofs the skin and hair.

**Seborrheic dermatitis.** Seborrheic dermatitis is a skin or scalp disorder with white scales and sometimes yellow flakes that cause the scalp or skin to itch (pruritus) and turn red. Sometimes, there are pustules (large fluid-filled, blisterlike areas) present on the scalp.

**Senescent baldness.** When hair thinning takes place in older men or women without a pattern, it is called *senescent baldness*. It is due to the thinning of the keratinocytes and is age-related. It can be diagnosed by ascertaining first that male-pattern baldness is not part of the family history and, second, that hair thinning, which became apparent after age 50, is due to thinning of the keratinocytes.

**Tissue.** The proliferated cells change from one cell to another and become differentiated into specialized cells that make up tissues and organs.

**Tissue types.** There are four main tissue types in the human body: *epithelial, connective, muscle,* and *nerve tissue.*

**Telogen.** Telogen is the phase in the hair growth cycle when 10% to 15% of the hair fibers are in a state of rest after the growing phase. The Telogen phase lasts from two to eight months, before the hair falls out. A hair fiber in the Telogen phase is also called a *club hair* due to the shape of the root of the Telogen hair. The root of the Telogen hair does not have a sheath, as shown in **Figure 4.19**.

**Telogen effluvium (TE).** If the number of hairs in the Telogen phase increases by more than 10% to 15% because of some shock to the system and, perhaps, even reaches as much as a 30% increase, excessive hair shedding will take place, resulting in temporary hair loss. However, new hair continues to grow; that is the reason why this type of hair loss is temporary.

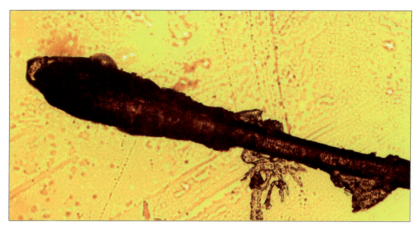

Figure 4.19. The Telogen hair root is club-shaped and without a sheath. This sample was taken from the front of the head of a 29-year-old patient who was losing his hair in that area. Photo courtesy of Avlon® Research Center.

**Traction alopecia (TA).** The hair loss experienced around the temple area due to braids, ponytails, weaves, or locks is called *traction alopecia*. The hair is pulled back with high tension and kept in this position sometimes for weeks. Due to trauma to the hair follicle, the hair loss or traction alopecia takes place. Traction alopecia can thus also be called *traumatic alopecia*.

**Transepidermal water loss (TEWL).** Measuring the TEWL of the skin is an important noninvasive method of assessing the efficiency of the skin as a protective barrier. The loss of water through the epidermis relates to the barrier function of the skin. The measurement of epidermal (skin) water loss is based on the vapor gradient (or open-chamber) principle. The open-chamber design maintains the free natural evaporation from the surface with minimal impact on the skin being examined.

Two sets of temperature/humidity sensors are mounted in a measurement chamber at different heights above the skin surface. The measurement chamber is open to allow the skin to "breathe" freely, and the evaporation rate follows Fick's law of diffusion. The displayed reading is called *transepidermal water loss* (TEWL) and expressed in units of g/$m^2$/h.

**Trichogram.** A photographic method called *phototrichogram* is used to quantify the ratio of Anagen and Telogen hair on 1 cm$^2$ of the scalp. The person's hair is shaved off of 1 cm$^2$ of the scalp. The photographs are taken on Day 0 and Day 2. The fibers in the Anagen phase grow longer than those in the Telogen phase. The number of Anagen and Telogen hairs are counted and the ratio of Anagen:Telogen hairs becomes a benchmark for determining the growth rate.

**Vertex**. The vertex is the backside of the top, or the crown, of the head. Many women start to lose their hair in the back of the crown area of the head, which then expands to the frontal middle of the head.

## References

Abell, E. (1988). Histologic response to topically applied minoxidil in male pattern alopecia. *Clinics in Dermatology, 6*(4), 192–194.

Aldosary, B. M., Sutter, M. E., Schwartz, M., & Morgan, B. W. (2012). Case series of selenium toxicity from a nutritional supplement. *Clinical Toxicology, 50*, 5–64.

Baden, H. P., & Kubilus, J. (1983). Effect of minoxidil on cultured keratinocytes. *Journal of Investigative Dermatology, 81*(6), 558–560.

Bent, S., Kane, C., Shinohara, K., Neuhaus, J., Hudes, E. S., Goldberg, H., & Avins, A. L. (2006). Saw palmetto for benign prostatic hyperplasia. *New England Journal of Medicine, 35*(6), 557–566.

Beoy, L. A., Eoei, W. J., & Hay, Y. K. (2010). Effects of tocotrienol supplementation on hair growth in human volunteers. *Tropical Life Science Research, 21*(20), 9–99.

Bergfeld, W. F. (1998). Retinoids and hair growth. *Journal of the American Academy Dermatology, 39*(2), S86–S89.

Bernard, B. A. (2005). The hair follicle: Structure and function. In Bouillon & Wilkinson (Eds.), *The science of hair care* (2nd ed, pp. 67–81). Boca Raton, FL: CRC Taylor & Francis.

Cardin, C. (1998). Isolated dandruff. In Baran & Maibach (Eds.), *Textbook of cosmetic dermatology* (2nd ed., pp. 193–200). London, UK: Martin Dunitz.

Clark, R. V., Hermann, D. J., Cunningham, G .R., Wilson, T .H., Morrill, B .B., & Hobbs, S. (2004). Marked suppression of dihydrotestosterone in men with benign prostatic hyperplasia by dutasteride, a dual 5-a reductase inhibitor. *Journal of Clinical Endocrinology & Metabolism, 89*(5), 2179–2184.

Comben, N., Clark, R. J., & Sutherland, D. J. B. (1984). Clinical observations on the response of equine hoof defects to dietary supplementation with biotin. *The Veterinary Record, 115*, 642–645.

Conlon, I., & Raff, M. (1999). Size control in animal development. *Cell, 96*, 235–244.

Cormack, D. H. (2001). *Essential histology*. Hagerstown, MD: Lippincott, Williams, & Wilkins.

Courtois, M., Loussouarn, G., Hourseau, C., & Grollier, J. F. (1994). Hair cycle and alopecia. *Skin Pharmacology, 61*, 84–89.

Dargie, H.J., Dollery, C.T., & Daniel, J. (1977). Minoxidil in resistant hypertension. *Lancet, September 10*, 518.

Dhariwala, M. Y., & Ravikumar, P. (2019). An overview of herbal alternatives in androgenetic alopecia. *Journal of Cosmetic Dermatology, 18*, 966–975.

Draelos, Z. D. (2010). Antiaging ingredients. In M. Schlossman (Ed.), *The chemistry and manufacture of cosmetics: Cosmetic specialties and ingredients* (pp. 57–88). Carol Stream, IL: Allured Publishing.

Draelos, Z. D., & Pugliese, P. T. (2011). *Physiology of the skin* (3rd ed.). Carol Stream, IL: Allured Publishing.

Drake, L., Hordinsky, M., Fiedler, V., Swinehart, J., Unger, W. P., Cotteril, P. C., . . . & Waldstreicher, J. (1999). The effects of finasteride on scalp skin and serum androgen levels in men with androgenetic alopecia. *Journal of the American Academy of Dermatology, 41*(4), 550–554.

Dubief, C., Mellul, M., Loussouarn, G., & Saint-Léger, D. (2005). Hair care products. In Bouillon & Wilkinson (Eds.) *The science of hair care* (2nd ed., pp. 129–167). Boca Raton, FL: CRC Taylor & Francis.

Durusoy, C., Ozenli, Y., Adiguzel, A., Budakoglu, Y., Tugal, O., Arikan, S., . . . & Gulec, A. T. (2009). The role of psychological factors and serum zinc, folate and Vitamin B12 levels in the aetiology of trichodynia: a case-control study. *Clinical and Experimental Dermatology, 34*, 789–792.

Elewski, B. W. (2005). Clinical diagnosis of common scalp disorders. *Journal of Investigative Dermatology [Symposium Proceedings], 10*(3), 190–193.

Everts, H. B. (2012). Endogenous retinoids in the hair follicle and sebaceous gland. *Biochimica et Biophysica, 1821*, 222-229.

Ferry, J. J., Forbes, K. K., James, Vanderlugt, J. T., & Szpunar, G. J. (1990). Influence of tretinoin on the percutaneous absorption of minoxidil from an aqueous topical solution. *Clinical Pharmacology and Therapeutics, 47*(4), 439–446.

Friedman, E. S., Friedman, P. M., Cohen, D. E., & Washenik, K. (2002). Allergic contact dermatitis to topical minoxidil solution: Etiology and treatment. *Journal of the American Academy of Dermatology, 46*(2), 309–312.

Goldberg, L. J., & Lenzy, Y. (2010). Nutrition and hair. *Clinics in Dermatology, 28*, 412-419.

Guo, E. L., & Katta, R. (2017). Diet and hair loss: Effects of nutrient deficiency and supplement use. *Dermatology Practical & Conceptual, 7*(1), 1–10.

Gupta, M., & Mysore, V. (2016). Classifications of patterned hair loss: A review. *Journal of Cutaneous and Aesthetic Surgery, 9*(1), 3–12.

Habib, F. K., Ross, M., Ho, C. K. H., Lyons, V., & Chapman, K. (2005). Serenoa repens (Permixon®) inhibits the 5a-reductase activity of human prostate cancer cell lines without interfering with PSA expression. *International Journal of Cancer, 114*, 190-194.

Han, J. H., Kwon, O. S., Chung, J. J., Cho, K. H., Eun, H. C., & Kim K. H. (2004). Effect of minoxidil on proliferation and apoptosis in dermal papilla cells of human hair follicle. *Journal of Dermatological Science, 34*, 91–98.

Hocker, H. (2002). Fiber morphology. In Simpson & Crawshaw (Eds.), *Wool: Science and technology* (pp. 60–79). Cambridge, England: Woodhead.

Hsu, S. (2005). Green tea and the skin. *Journal of the American Academy of Dermatology, 52*(6), 1049–1059.

Jacobs, B., & Buttigieg, C.F. (1981). Minoxidil: Six years' experience in Australia. *Medical Journal of Australia, 1*, 477.

Jacomb, R.G., & Brunnberg, F.J. (1976). The use of minoxidil in the treatment of severe essential hypertension: a report on 100 patients. *Clinical Science and Molecular Medicine, 51*, 579S–581S.

Joshi, R. S. (2011). The inner root sheath and the men associated with it eponymically. *International Journal of Tricology, 3*(1), 57–62.

Kenekura, T., Yotsumoto, S., Maeno, N., Kamenosono, A., Saruwatari, H., Uchino, Y., . . . & Kanzaki, T. (2005). Selenium deficiency: Report of a case. *Clinical & Experimental Dermatology, 30*, 346–348.

Khumalo, N. P., & Ngwanya, R. M. (2006). Traction alopecia: 2 % topical minoxidil shows promise: Report of two cases. *Journal of the European Academy of Dermatology and Venereology, 21*, 433–434.

Kligman, A. M. (1988). The comparative histopathology of male-pattern baldness and senescent baldness. *Clinics in Dermatology, 6*(4), 108–118.

Levin, O. L., & Behrman, H. T. (1946). *Your hair and its care*. New York, NY: Emerson Books.

Lewallen, R., Francis, S., Fisher, B., Richards, J., Li, J., Dawson, T., . . . & McMichael, A. (2015). Hair care practices and structural evaluation of scalp and hair shaft parameters in African-American and Caucasian women. *Journal of Cosmetic Dermatology, 14*, 216–223.

Light, D. B. (2009). *Cells, tissues, and skin*. New York, NY: Chelsea House.

Limat, A., Suormala, T., Hunziker, T., Waelti, E. R., Braathen, L. R., & Baumgartner, R. (1996). Proliferation and differentiation of cultured human follicular keratinocytes are not influenced by biotin. *Archives of Dermatology Research*, 31–38.

Loussouarn, G. (2001). African hair growth parameters. *British Journal of Dermatology, 145*, 294–297.

MacDonald, R., Tacklind, J. W., Rutks, I., & Wilt, T. J. (2012). Serenoa repens monotherapy for benign prostate hyperplasia (BPH): An updated Cochrane systematic review. *British Journal of Urology International*, 1756–1761.

McCray, M. K., & Roenigk, H. H. (1983). Cosmetic correction of alopecia. *American Family Physician, 28*(4), 207.

McMichael, A. J. (2003). Hair and scalp disorders in ethnic populations. *Dermatologic Clinics, 21*, 629–644.

Nicholson, A. G., Harland, C., Bull, R. H., Mortimer, P. S., & Cook, M. G. (1993). Chemically induced cosmetic alopecia. *British Journal of Dermatology, 128*, 537–541.

Olsen, E. A., Callender, V., Sperling, L., McMichael, A., Anstrom, K. J., Bergfeld, W., . . . & Whiting, D. A. (2008). Central scalp alopecia photographic scale in African-American women. *Dermatologic Therapy, 21*, 264–267.

Ozcelik, D. (2005). Extensive traction alopecia attributable to ponytail hairstyle and its treatment with hair transplantation. *Aesthetic Plastic Surgery, 29*, 325–327.

Park, H., Kim, C. W., Kim, S. S., & Park, C. W. (2009). The therapeutic effect and the changed serum zinc level after zinc supplementation in alopecia areata patients who had a low serum zinc level. *Annals of Dermatology, 21*(2), 142-146.

Pennisi, A. J., Singsen, B. H., Ettenger, R. B., & Hanson, V. H. (1977). Minoxidil therapy in children with severe hypertension. *The Journal of Pediatrics, 90*(5), 813-819

Pierard-Franchimont, C., De Donker, P., Cauwenbergh, & Pierard, G. E. (1998). Ketoconazole shampoo: Effect of long-term use in androgenetic alopecia. *Dermatology, 196*, 474–477.

Prager, N., Bickett, K., French, N., & Marcovici, G. (2002). A randomized, double blind, placebo-controlled trial to determine the effectiveness of botanically derived inhibitors of 5AR in the treatment of androgenetic alopecia. *The Journal of Alternative and Complimentary Medicine, 8*(2), 1–20.

Pyo, H. K., Yoo, H. G., Won, C. H., Lee, S. H., Kang, Y. J., Eun, H. C., , , , & Kim, K. H. (2007), The effect of tripeptide-copper complex on human hair growth in vitro. *Archives of Pharmacologic Research, 30*(7), 834–839.

Rasheed, H., Mahgoub, Hegazy, R., El-Komy, M., Hay R. A., Hamid, M. A., & Hamdy, E. (2013). Serum ferritin and vitamin D in female hair loss: do they play a role? *Skin Pharmacology and Physiology, 26*, 101-107.

Robbins, C. R. (2002). *Chemical and physical behavior of human hair* (4th ed.). New York, NY: Springer.

Roenigk, H. H. (1998). Hair loss: Surgical treatments. In Baran & Maibach (Eds.), *Textbook of cosmetic dermatology* (2nd ed., pp. 633–642). London, UK: Martin Dunitz.

Rogers, N. E., & Avram, M. R. (2008). Medical treatments for male- and female-pattern hair loss. *Journal of the American Academy of Dermatology, 59*(4), 547–566.

Rushton, D. H., Norris, M. J., Dover, R., & Busuttil. (2002). Causes of hair loss and the developments in hair rejuvenation. *International Journal of Cosmetic Science, 24*, 17–23.

Savin, R. C. (1992). A method for visually describing and quantitating hair loss in male-pattern baldness. *Journal of Investigative Dermatology, 9*, 604.

Shai, A., Maibachi, H. I., & Baran, R. (2002). *Handbook of cosmetic skin care*. London, UK: Martin Dunitz.

Shin, H. S., Won, C. H., Lee, S. H., Kwon, O. S., Kim, K. H., & Eun, H. C. (2007). *American Journal of Clinical Dermatology, 8*(5), 285–290.

Syed, A. N., Syed M. N., & Mathew, J. (2022). Texture Talk: Reinforcing Curly Hair Health. *Cosmetics & Toiletries Magazine, 137* (2), 46-56.

Thibaut, S., Barbarat, P., Leroy, F., & Bernard, B. A. (2007). Human hair keratin network and curvature. *International Journal of Dermatology, 46*(S1), 7–10.

Thomas, J. (2005). Androgenetic alopecia: Current status. Indian *Journal of Dermatology, 50*(4), 179–190.

Trachy, R. E., Fors, T. D., Pickart, L. & Uno, H. (1991). The hair follicle-stimulating properties of peptide copper complexes: Results in C3H mice. *Annals of the New York Academy of Sciences*, 468–469.

Trost, L. B., Bergfeld, W. F., & Calogeras, E. (2006). The diagnosis and treatment of iron deficiency and its potential relationship to hair loss. *Journal of the American Academy of Dermatology, 54*(5), 824–844.

Vazquez, B., Avila, G., Segura, D., & Escalante, B. (1996). Anti-inflammatory activity of extracts from aloe vera gel. *Journal of Ethnopharmacology, 55*, 69–75.

Veyrac, G., Chiffoleau, A., Baily, C., Baudot, S., Beaudouin, S., & Larousse, C. (1995). Cutaneous application of minoxidil during pregnancy: Hairy infant. *Therapie, 50*(5), 474–476.

Whiting, D. A. (1999). Traumatic alopecia. *International Journal of Dermatology, 38*(S1), 34–44.

Wojciech, P., Ross, M. W., & Gordon, K. I. (2003). *Histology: A text and atlas with cell and molecular biology*. Hagerstown, MD: Lippincott, Williams & Wilkins.

# CHAPTER 5

# Cleansing the Hair & Scalp

Humans have been cleansing their hair, scalp, and body from millenia. As early as 4000 B.C., Eurasians managed to cleanse their hair and body in bathhouses (Smith, 2007, p. 45). In Mesopotamia, personal cleanliness had become a common occurrence, by 3000 B.C. (p. 46).

The cosmetics business was thriving in Egypt in the ancient world, as the Egyptians harvested domestic vegetable source materials such as lotus flowers and other sudsing plants for cleanliness and washing of the hair and body. The early Egyptians, Sumerians, Orientals, Romans and modern-day Jews, Christians, Muslims, and Hindus made religious and hygienic rituals out of bathing and cleansing the hair (Schlossman, 2006, p. 739). In the 20th century, bathing became an achievable and convenient chore at home for the common man.

The ancient Indians and the ancient Chinese used semicrushed natural reetha shells in boiled water, which were cooled before using for cleansing the hair and body. Reetha is a Sanskrit word for soap berries. When reetha shells became popular, they were exported to Middle Eastern regions and, finally, to Europe through trade routes. When they arrived in Europe, they were renamed with the Latin name *Sap indus*, where sap means soap and indus means from India.

Reetha is still very popular in India, Pakistan, Bangladesh, and China. Lately, with the advent of the natural movement in the United States and Europe, reetha has become a significantly popular ingredient, readily-available for purchase in physical as well as virtual marketplaces. Various U.S. hair brands have added reetha extract to shampoos as an additive. There is a need for more research regarding reetha's cleansing ability and impact on the moisture of the hair, and its impact on the TEWL, moisture, and erythema of the scalp.

In the 19th and earlier centuries, soap was a favored product for cleansing the hair and body. A soap is defined as the salt of an alkali (base) and a fatty acid. Soaps are basic in pH, pH > 10. In the United States, very early shampoos were made from liquid coconut oil soap. These soap-based shampoos lathered more quickly and superbly than bar soaps, rinsed easily from the hair, and performed better in hard water in terms of their foam (Markland, 1975, p. 1283).

By the middle of the 20th century, shampoos and bubble baths were introduced in the form of liquid products that contained synthetic detergents, which were closer to the pH of hair and skin, $4 < pH < 6.5$. Since then, detergent-based products have become products for everyday use. There have been numerous innovations in the area of shampoos and cleansing products in the last century and they are continuing to this day.

According to one estimate, the sale of shampoos reached US$ 29.38 billion in 2019 and is projected to reach US$ 39.27 billion by 2027 globally. Some of the reasons for this growth are hair problems among millennials and also other unmet needs of color-treated and textured hair with regard to ease of combing and dry scalp. Also, the spread of COVID-19 has increased the demand for shampoos in order to keep the hair and scalp clear of microbial contamination (Fortune Business Insights, 2019).

Some of the newest innovations in shampoos in the last two decades have been shampoos containing apple cider, caffeine for stimulating the scalp, shampoos for retaining color in color-treated hair, purple shampoos for removing brassy tones from blonde hair, and a cleansing conditioner also known as CoWash (Conditioning Wash) for curly and coily hair types.

Thus, cleansing of hair is an important category, and a great deal of attention needs to be given to the science of shampoos for all hair types, straight, wavy, curly and coily. Since research has shown that the hair structure and the scalp associated with straight vs curly/coily hair are different, these differences must be kept in mind when designing cleansing products.

## The Purpose of Cleansing Products & Shampoos

An abundance of sebum-secreting sebaceous glands can be found underneath the human scalp. Each hair follicle is surrounded by one or more sebaceous glands. There are at least as many sebaceous glands as there are hairs on the human head, ~100,000 to 150,000 hairs. The face may have as many as 400 to 900 sebaceous glands per square centimeter (Smith & Thiboutot, 2008, p. 271).

Sebum is a sticky, oily substance. Various scientists have already conducted a great deal of chemical analysis of sebum, showing that sebum contains triglycerides (35%), free fatty acids (20%), wax and cholesterol esters (19%), squalene (11%), free cholesterol (9%), and paraffins (6%; Wong, 1997, p. 34). On a regular basis, sebum is first secreted from a sebaceous gland in the human scalp. Then, this sebum travels along the hair shaft, from the root of the hair fiber to the tip. The secreted sebum also transfers from one fiber to adjacent hair fibers.

Along with sebum transfer, environmental factors such as pollution, humidity, and dust deposit make cleansing the hair and scalp necessary on a regular basis. In addition, the scalp turns over its cells abundantly in many individuals. These cells accumulate as debris on the scalp in the form of a film. Underneath this film, moisture and sebum help proliferate various bacteria and a fungus belonging to the *Malassezia species*. This microbial proliferation leads to the formation of sticky, white to yellow flakes on the scalp, and in some cases scalp itching. Individuals suffering from this scalp itch, scratch the scalp with their fingernails and injure the scalp.

The scalp, face, and ears have more sebaceous glands than the rest of the skin and thus become oilier. This is known as seborrhea, which predisposes individuals to the development of seborrheic dermatitis. The symptoms of seborrheic dermatitis are red, scaly patches all over the scalp and body (Smith & Thiboutot, 2008, p. 271). Therefore, it is necessary to remove excess sebum, fungus, and bacteria from the surface of the scalp and body on a regular basis.

## Hair & Scalp Cleansing Practices of Caucasians & African-Americans

According to Lewallen (2015), 63% of individuals in the U.S. cleanse their hair every two days, and 27% cleanse daily (p. 219). This habit may result in overcleansing of the hair and scalp. By contrast, the sebaceous glands of African-descent individuals are not as active and produce less sebum. According to this study, 50% of African-descent consumers cleanse their hair every two weeks, and 40% cleanse their hair every week, on average. A new segment of consumers with wavy or curly hair has emerged within the Caucasian consumer category. These consumers with wavy hair (Types 2, 3A, and 3B) have indicated that they do not shampoo their hair every day but every three or four days. Also, they have noticed that their hair requires lightly foaming cleansers or conditioners, as they do not have excessive sebum production. This new concept has given birth to a new category of cleansing product called Co-Wash, that is, washing hair with conditioners. In the past, most consumers equated cleansing of the hair with abundant foam or lather, however scientific research has shown that low-foaming or non-foaming emulsifiers can achieve excellent cleansing as well. In this latest movement, both African-Americans and curly-haired Caucasians, use low-foaming conditioners for cleansing reguarly and only incorporate a high foaming shampoo every three to four weeks into their regimen.

## Differences in Hair & Scalp By Hair Type & Ethnicity

Before discussing the attributes of hair after shampoo use, it is important to note the differences in Type 1, Type 3, and Type 4 hair and scalp. Type 1 (Caucasian) hair is straight and has the lowest ellipticity, as compared to Types 3 and 4 (mixed ethnicity and African-descent) hair

(Syed, Ventura, & Syed, 2013, p. 259). The lower ellipticity of hair connotes that the hair fiber is more uniform, or cylindrical, and has fewer variations in diameter along its shaft, whereas high ellipticity means the fibers are not uniform and vary significantly in their diameter along the length of the hair fiber. Higher ellipticity fibers are curly (Type 3) and curly-to-coily (Type 4) and, consequently, difficult to comb. Fibers with higher ellipticity are weaker in their tensile strength, as compared to fibers that possess low ellipticity. Type 1 hair displays ellipticity values of 1.0-1.40, while Type 4 hair displays higher ellipticity values of 1.0-3.25. Wet African-descent (Type 4) hair is 23 times more difficult to comb than wet Caucasian (Type 1) hair (Syed & Syed, 2017, p. 21). Dry African-descent (Type 4) hair is 32 times more difficult to comb, as compared to dry Caucasian (Type 1) hair. Thus, wet Type 4 hair is ~47% weaker than wet Type 1 hair. Similarly, dry Type 4 hair is 26% weaker than dry Type 1 hair (Syed et al., 1995, p. 48). Wet hair is generally weaker than dry hair. These results indicate that considerable care and caution should be exercised when combing wet Types 3 and 4 hair, as compared to Type 1 hair.

Studies comparing skin properties by ethnicity are not conclusive. One study comparing the skin of African-Americans with that of Caucasians reported that the two types of skin are not different with respect to skin moisture, transepidermal water loss (TEWL), and Doppler Velocimetry (LVD) (Berardesca & Maibach, 1988, p. 65). Another study by Syed, et al., (2022) showed differences in TEWL values of African-American versus Caucasian scalps. The TEWL values of African-American scalps tended to be higher than those of Caucasian scalps (p. 50).

## Impact of Detergents on Hair & Scalp Integrity

Detergents are surfactants (surface-active agents) with cleansing properties when used in dilute solutions. Surfactants are materials that reduce the surface tension between two phases, be it two liquids, a liquid and a gas, or a liquid and a solid. For many decades, most shampoo formulations were developed mainly with the detergent sodium lauryl sulfate (SLS) to cleanse the hair and scalp. Shampoos formulated with harsh detergents such as sodium lauryl sulfate or ammonium lauryl sulfate (ALS) strip the hair of its F layer, some amount of CMC between the cuticle layers, and the CMC of the innermost cuticle layer and the cortical cells. Sandhu and Robbins (1993) conducted experiments where they immersed and shook hair fibers alternately in 5% solutions of SLS and ALS for 4 hours and, then, determined the amount of proteins in the water. The results indicated that SLS and ALS dissolved most proteins from the hair, compared to water as a control (p. 172).

When African-American and Caucasian skin was exposed to a solution of 0.5% and 2.0% SLS, a common ingredient in shampoos, the two skin types showed a significant difference in terms of TEWL, moisture content, and LDV (Berardesca & Maibach, 1988, p. 67). African-American skin had significantly higher TEWL after treatment with both 0.5% and 2.0% solutions. The water content of African-American skin was also low when treated with the two solutions. When the lipids were removed from African-American skin and Caucasian skin, African-American skin had very high TEWL values for both solutions of SLS. The 2% SLS solution increased TEWL significantly, as compared to 0.5% SLS (p. 69). Thus, it was inferred that African-American skin is very susceptible to sodium lauryl sulfate in shampoos.

When the irritation of 0.5% SLS was tested on menstrual women on Day 1 and Days 9 to 11, it was found that women on Day 1 of the menstrual cycle reacted more strongly than on Days 9 to 11 in terms of skin irritation, using TEWL and visual scoring at $p < .05$ (Agner, Damm, & Skouby, 1991, p. 566). Elsner, Wilhelm, and Maibach (1991) found that SLS produced skin irritation in pre- and postmenstrual women, but this response decreased with age (p. 77). Therefore, the type and concentration of detergents should be carefully decided while keeping in mind the health of women in terms of long-term skin and scalp moisture and irritation.

Mizutani et al. (2016) explained the mechanism of rough skin from exposure to SLS and came to the conclusion that even small concentrations (50 μg/mL) of SLS stimulated the generation of reactive oxygen species (ROS) through the interaction with the cell membrane of the epidermis, producing damaged and rough skin (p. 999).

Another study on Japanese skin showed that a 5.0% solution of sodium dodecyl sulfate (SDS) induced chapping and scaling of the stratum corneum (SC) and a significant decrease in water retention (Imokawa, Akasaki, Minematsu, & Kawai, 1989, p. 45). The lipids were depleted from the intercellular spaces of the stratum corneum, and these lipids contained cholesterol, cholesterol esters, free fatty acids, and sphingolipids. Effendy and Maibach (1996, p. 19) compared the skin irritation caused by detergents, using TEWL as an evaluator, and found the ranking of detergents in terms of their TEWL as follows:

Increasing TEWL ↑
- Linear alkyl ($C_{12}$) sulfonate
- Sodium lauryl sulfate
- Sodium laureth sulfate
- Polysorbate 20

The TEWL ranking for 7.0% solutions was as follows:

Sodium lauryl sulfate > Cocamidopropyl betaine (CAPB)

Thus, TEWL rankings can be used as a helpful tool in selecting the gentlest detergents for shampoos that will keep the scalp healthy in terms of its stratum corneum and moisture-holding capacity.

Most studies on SLS are based on low concentrations of SLS and their impact on skin TEWL, pH, and moisture using bioengineering techniques. Faucher and Goddard (1978) studied the interaction of SLS with skin at actual use levels of 10% to 15% SLS in shampoos and found that the amount of sodium lauryl sulfate absorbed by the stratum corneum was almost linear to its concentration (p. 329). However, the absorption of SLS decreased when nonionic detergents such as $C_{11-15}$Pareth-9 were included in the formulation (p. 333).

Most of the literature is concentrated on studying the impact of sodium lauryl sulfate on the skin. However, marketplace shampoos use many different types of detergents for cleansing purposes. Therefore, there is a need to compare various detergents utilized commonly in shampoos. One such study was conducted by the author of this book in 2008, where commonly used detergents in shampoos at 15% concentration in water were tested with respect to their effect on skin. TEWL values were measured for seven to eight subjects (Syed, Hussain, & Hussain, 2008, p. 39).

The TEWL values for these detergents were then compared and ranked using statistical techniques such as ANOVA Tukey B tests. Shown here is the final detergent ranking from lowest to highest TEWL:

Disodium laureth sulfosuccinate

Ammonium laureth sulfate

Sodium laureth sulfate

Ammonium cocoyl isethionate

Cocoamidopropyl amine oxide

Disodium cocoamphodipropionate

Cocomidopropyl hydoxysultaine

Lauramide DEA

Sodium cocoyl isethionate

Polysorbate 80

Sodium lauroyl sarcosinate

Ammonium lauryl sulfate

Sodium lauryl sulfate

Sodium $C_{12}$-$C_{14}$ olefin sulfonate

↓ Increasing TEWL

## Mitigating Deleterious Effects of Sodium Lauryl Sulfate on the Skin

Mizutani et al. (2016) postulated that SLS stimulates the generation of a reactive oxygen species (ROS) through interaction with the cell membrane of the epidermis. To combat this oxidation process oatmeal extract was utilized. When 20% oatmeal extract was applied to the skin, Mizutani et al. modulated the SLS-induced skin irritation, thereby confirming that they prevented the alteration of the cutaneous barrier (Vie et al., 2002, p. 124).

Huang and Chang (2008) studied the deleterious effects of SLS as a detergent on skin and found that, as deduced from various earlier studies,

SLS irritates the skin and disturbs the lipids of the stratum corneum. In this study, Ceramides 1 and 3 were applied from a cream vehicle, and the TEWL values were studied for 28 days. The researchers concluded that a combination of Ceramide 1 and 3 at 0.02% each reduced the TEWL values and increased skin hydration at $p < .05$ (p. 818). Therefore, to mitigate the negative effects of SLS on the skin or scalp, ceramides may be incorporated in formulations such as creams and shampoos to maintain a healthy scalp.

## Evolution of Detergents in Cleansing Products, Types of Detergents, & Their Impact on Hair & Scalp

The word *shampoo* is derived from the Hindi word *champo*, which means massaging or squeezing (Beauquey, 2005, p. 83). A shampoo is a liquid, gel, or cream, utilizing surface-active materials capable of removing dirt or grime from the surface of the hair and scalp while producing foam during application and massage.

Early shampoos contained soaps that were prepared by neutralizing fats or oils with lyes such as sodium or potassium hydroxides. These shampoos generally had alkaline pH in the range of 10.0-10.5. These soaps, in the liquid form, were not very effective in cleansing the hair and scalp in the presence of hard water. Generally, hard water contains calcium and magnesium ions and precipitates the soap into calcium/magnesium stearates, which are water insoluble and stick to the scalp. These soap-based shampoos rendered the hair alkaline and dull, leaving behind a film of soap on the hair and scalp surface. If the hair is rendered alkaline, the cuticles open, the hair is weaker in terms of its elasticity, and the scalp is compromised. Therefore, it is always desirable not to alter the natural pH of the hair and scalp during the cleansing process. A pH of 5.0-5.8 is more favorable for the normal apathogenic resident flora; hence, a healthy scalp (Schmid-Wendtner & Korting, 2007, p. 43).

Since the mid-20th century, a new class of cleansing agents has been synthesized that gained popularity over soap-based cleansing products. These new shampoos were high-foaming, performed very well in hard water, and left the hair surface squeaky clean, all without imparting a dull film on the surface of the hair and scalp.

# Classification of Detergents

Detergents can be categorized into five main classes: anionic, cationic, amphoteric, non-ionic, and natural detergents. Anionic detergents carry a negative charge, whereas cationic detergents carry a positive charge. Amphoteric detergents carry both positive and negative charges, while non-ionic detergents carry no charge.

## Anionic Detergents

Most of the detergents that are employed in shampoos in appreciable amounts are anionic in nature. Anionic detergents are negatively charged molecules that produce a rich and dense foam. Commonly used anionic detergents are divided into several groups according to their chemical structure: sulfates, sulfonates, sulfosuccinates, acyl isethionates, acyl taurates/taurides, carboxylates that are derived from amino acids, and carboxylates that are non-amino acid based.

### Group 1A: Sulfates

Sulfated detergents consist of alkyl sulfates and ethoxylated alkyl sulfates. The general structure of an alkyl sulfate and an ethoxylated sulfate is shown in **Figure 5.1** and **Figure 5.2** respectively. They are prepared by the sulfation of fatty alcohols, such as lauryl alcohol. Detergents in this group are sodium lauryl sulfate, ammonium lauryl sulfate, TEA-lauryl sulfate, sodium laureth sulfate, ammonium laureth sulfate, and TEA-laureth sulfate. Sodium lauryl sulfate is widely used in shampoos, but it impacts

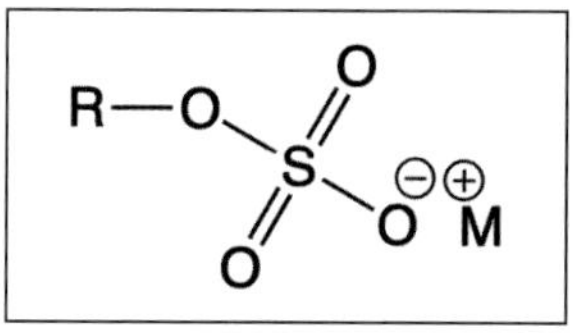

Figure 5.1. Structure of an alkyl sulfate, where $M^+$ is a cation that could be sodium, ammonium, or triethanolamine. R denotes alkyl group.

the stratum corneum of the skin negatively by increasing the TEWL of the skin, at $p < .05$. Ammonium lauryl sulfate also increases the TEWL of the skin significantly, at $p < .05$. Therefore, the use of sulfates in superior quality shampoos has significantly decreased over the last decade.

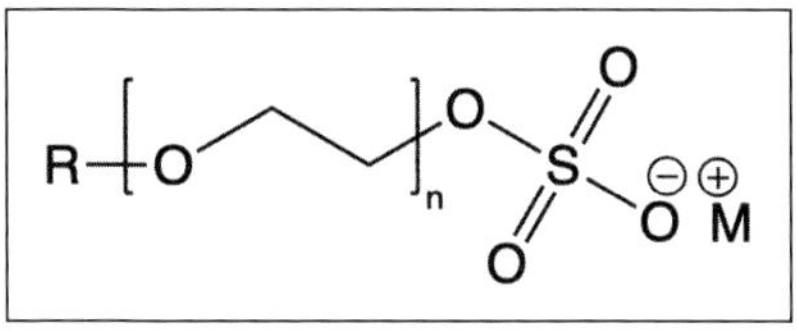

**Figure 5.2.** Structure of an ethoxylated alkyl sulfate, where $M^+$ is a cation that could be sodium, ammonium, or triethanolamine. R denotes alkyl group. The subscript n denotes the degree of ethoxylation.

### Group 1B: Sulfonates

The most widely used sulfonate is sodium $C_{14-16}$ olefin sulfonate (see **Figure 5.3** for structure), which is produced by sulfonating α-olefin with sulfuric anhydride. It is a harsh detergent in terms of its impact on the stratum corneum of the scalp, as it increases the TEWL of the skin significantly, $p = .008$, which is $< .05$ (Syed et al., 2008, p. 34 ).

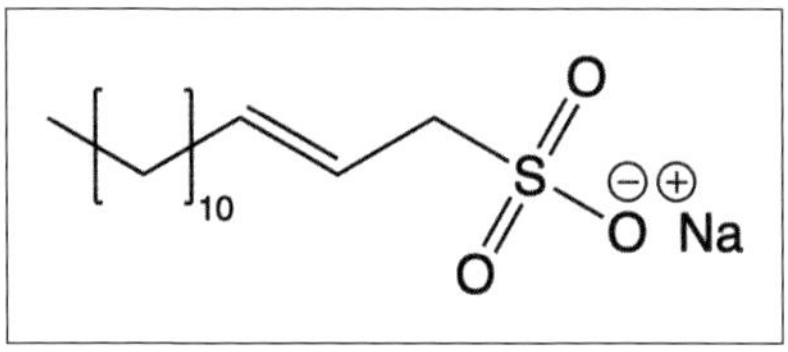

**Figure 5.3.** Structure of sodium $C_{14-16}$ olefin sulfonate.

### Group 1C: Sulfosuccinates

Sulfosuccinates are produced by a process in which (1) one of the carboxylic acid groups of sulfosuccinic acid is esterified with an alkyl alcohol, and (2) the second carboxylic acid group and the sulfonic group are neutralized by sodium or ammonium hydroxide. The structure of a common sulfosuccinate, disodium alkyl sulfosuccinate, is shown in **Figure 5.4**.

Alkyl sulfosuccinates are ethoxylated to make them milder to the skin, where the alkyl chain is ethoxylated with 2 or 3 moles of ethylene oxide. Disodium laureth sulfosuccinate is significantly milder to the stratum corneum of the skin, $p = .01$, which is $< .05$ (Syed et al., 2008, p. 34). The structure of disodium or diammonium laureth sulfosuccinate is shown in **Figure 5.5**.

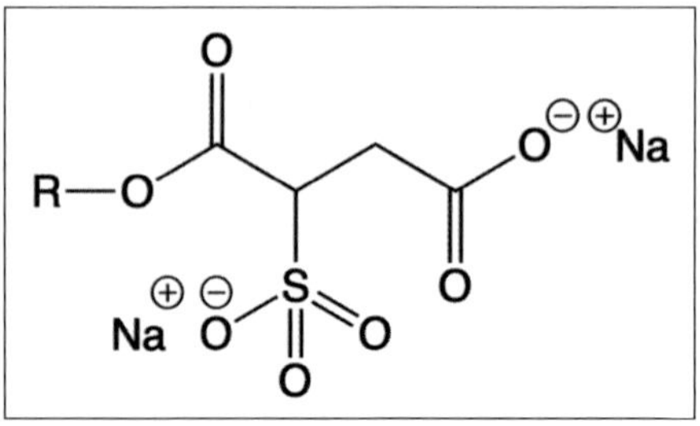

**Figure 5.4.** Structure of disodium alkyl sulfosuccinate, where R denotes alkyl group.

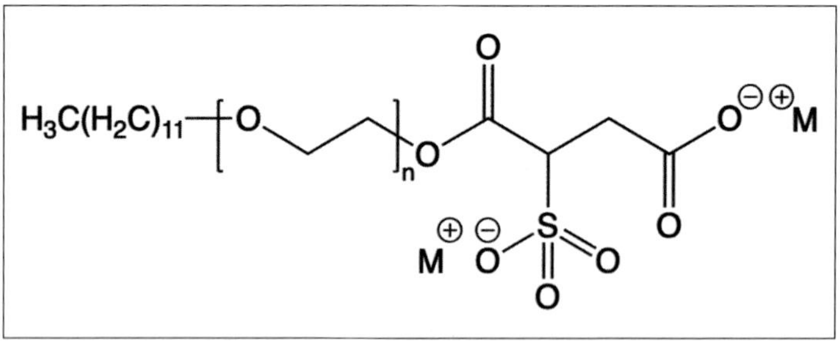

**Figure 5.5.** Structure of disodium or diammonium laureth sulfosuccinate, where M is the cation, $Na^+$ or $NH_4^+$ respectively. The subscript n denotes the degree of ethoxylation, where n averages between 1 and 4.

### Group 1D: Acyl Isethionates

Acyl isethionates were one of the first synthetic detergents on the market, available under the trade name *Igepons*. They are produced by a process in which first isethionic acid is combined with an acyl group; then, the acid group is neutralized with an alkali or ammonium hydroxide; hence, the name *acyl isethionate*. These detergents are also considered mild to the skin; however, they are poorly water soluble. For example, sodium cocoyl isethionate does not dissolve in water; thus, it is very difficult to dissolve it in a shampoo formulation. However, it is possible to dissolve sodium cocoyl isethionate in either self-emulsifying wax or amphoteric detergents such as disodium cocoamphodipropionate (Sun et al., 2003, pp. 566, 562). Ammonium cocoyl isethionate comes as a 30% solution in water and readily combines with other detergents in the formulations. Although this class of detergents is considered mild to the skin, it can dry the hair and skin if used at high concentrations. Ammonium cocoyl isethionate is not readily available commercially, but it is gentler to the skin than sodium cocoyl isethionate, $p < .05$ (Syed et al., 2008, p. 34). The structure of this class of compounds is depicted in **Figure 5.6**.

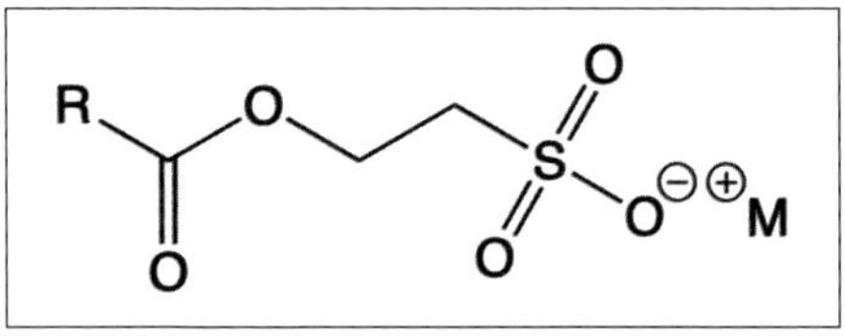

Figure 5.6. Structure of an acyl isethionate.

### Group 1E: Acyl Taurates or Taurides

The structure of taurates or taurides includes a hydrophilic head group that consists of N-methyltaurine, shown in **Figure 5.7**. The lipophilic group is then linked at the nitrogen site. The lipophilic group is usually a type of fatty acid. The cation is usually sodium however can also be potassium, calcium, or magnesium, etc. This class of detergents produces foam rapidly and with great volume, and is mild to the skin and scalp. The structure of sodium methyl acyl taurate is shown in **Figure 5.8**.

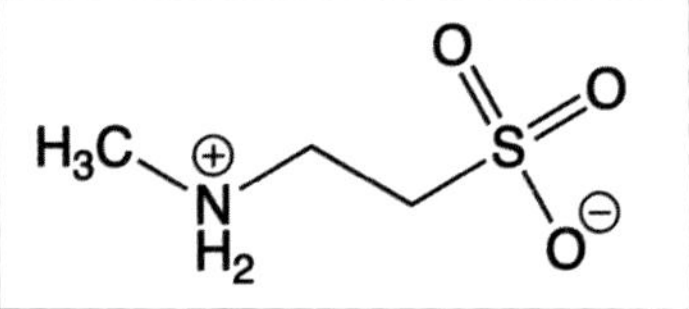

Figure 5.7. Structure of N-methyltaurine as a zwitterion.

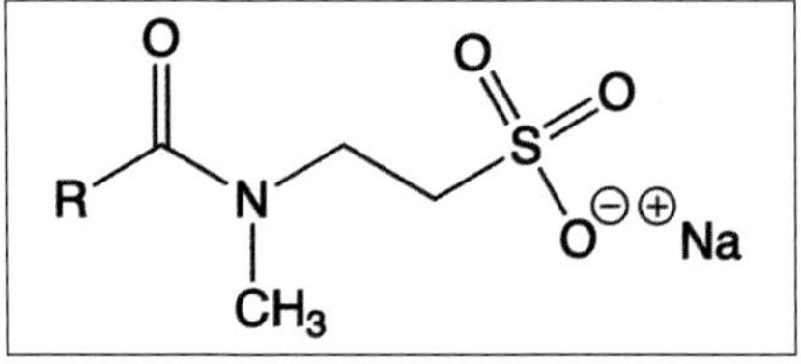

Figure 5.8. Structure of sodium methyl acyl taurate. Examples of the -RCO group are lauroyl, cocoyl, myristoyl, stearoyl, etc. The counterion is shown as sodium here but can be potassium, calcium, or magnesium, etc.

### Group 1F: Carboxylates (derived from amino acids)

Carboxylate detergents derived from amino acids such as sarcosine, glycine, or glutamic acid represent a milder class of detergents.

The structure of sarcosine, also known as *N*-methylglycine, is shown in **Figure 5.9**. Acyl groups are added to sarcosine at the amino site to produce *N*-acyl sarcosinate, whose structure is shown in **Figure 5.10**. These detergents are easily soluble in water and produce good foam, even in hard water. They are considered friendly to the skin, but data from Syed et al. (2008, p. 34) on TEWL values of the skin showed that sodium lauroyl sarcosinate at 15% is, actually, not mild to the skin, at $p < .001$.

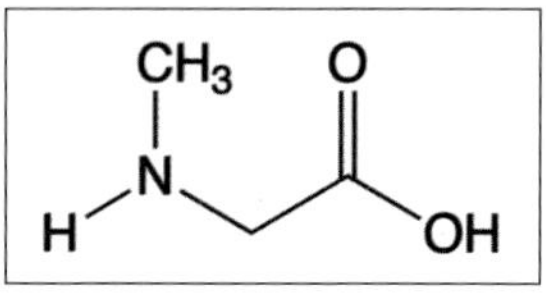

**Figure 5.9.** Structure of sarcosine.

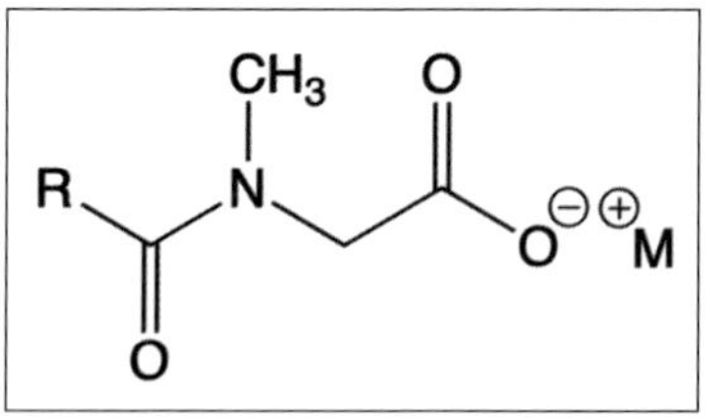

**Figure 5.10.** Structure of N-acyl sarcosinate. Examples of the -RCO group are lauroyl, cocoyl, etc. The cation may be sodium, potassium, or ammonium.

The amino acid glycine is the backbone of acyl glycinate detergents. The structures of glycine and N-acyl glycinate are shown in **Figure 5.11** and **Figure 5.12** respectively. Examples of acyl glycinates are potassium cocoyl glycinate, sodium cocoyl glycinate, and sodium lauroyl glycinate.

Shown in **Figure 5.13** is the structure of glutamic acid, which is an amino acid used to derive very mild detergents. For example, glutamic acid is used to synthesize sodium acyl glutamate (see **Figure 5.14** for structure). Examples of acyl glutamates are sodium cocoyl glutamate, sodium lauroyl glutamate, potassium cocoyl glutamate, and TEA-cocoyl glutamate.

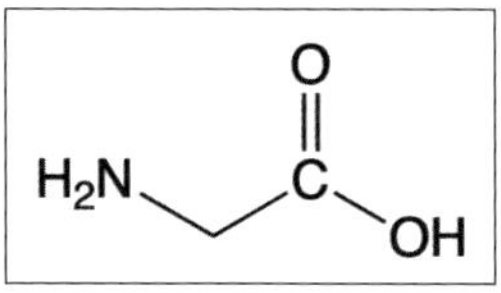

Figure 5.11. Structure of glycine.

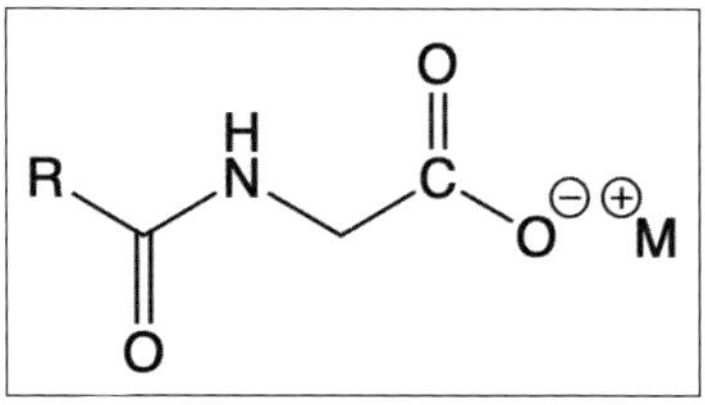

Figure 5.12. Structure of N-acyl glycinate. The most common -RCO groups are cocoyl and lauroyl. The cation may be sodium or potassium.

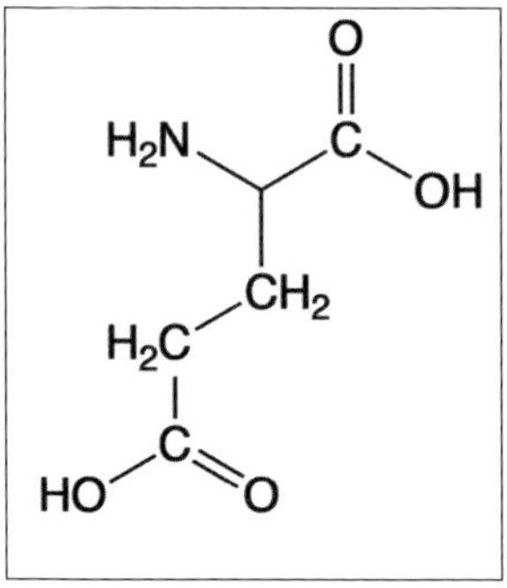

Figure 5.13. Structure of glutamic acid.

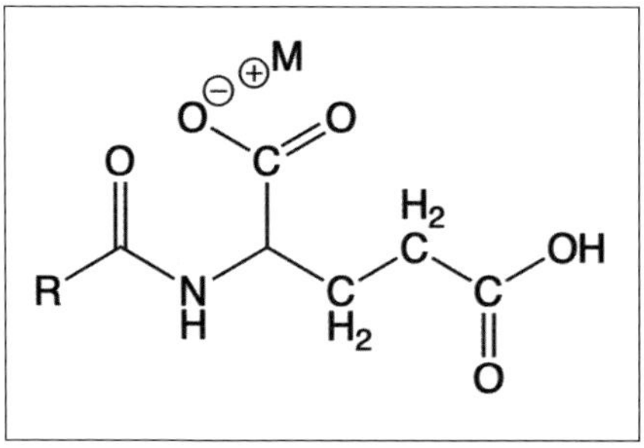

Figure 5.14. Structure of N-acyl glutamate. The most common -RCO groups are cocoyl and lauroyl. The cation may be sodium, potassium, or triethanolamine.

**Acylation of protein hydrolysates with fatty acid chlorides to produce acyl hydrolyzed proteins.** These are mixtures of lipid-based peptides of larger protein chains and lipid-based amino acids. One example of this type is potassium cocoyl hydrolyzed collagen. These protein-based cleansers are very gentle to the skin and are well-known for their conditioning properties for hair. They possess excellent power to disperse lime soap and can be used after products that may have left calcium or magnesium ions on the hair (Beauquey, 2005, p. 88). They do not foam well when compared to alkyl sulfates; however, they can be used in applications such as low-foaming mousses because of their conditioning properties.

### Group 1G: Carboxylates (non-amino acids)

Carboxylates are salts of ethoxylated fatty acid and thier general structure is shown in **Figure 5.15**. They are compatible with cationic polymers, which makes them good candidates for 2 in 1 detangling shampoos that contain anionic detergents such as alkyl sulfates and cationic detergents. One example of such a molecule is sodium trideceth-7 carboxylate. Referring to **Figure 5.15**, for sodium trideceth-7 carboxylate, the -R group is a tridecyl group ($-CH_2(CH_2)_{11}CH_3$), $n$ is on average 7, and $M$ is sodium.

Soaps represent another class of carboxylates as their structure consists of a fatty acid with a carboxyl group, neutralized with a sodium or potassium cation. It is well-known that soaps do not foam well, especially in hard water. Their solutions in water have a pH of $\approx 10$; therefore, they increase the pH of the skin or hair, leave a residue upon rinsing with water, and dry the hair and skin.

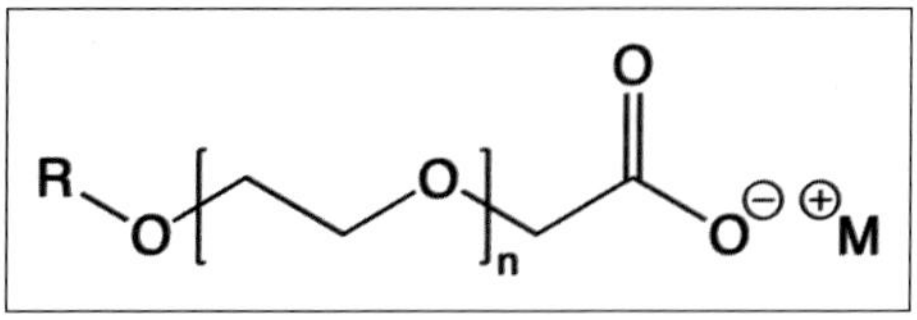

Figure 5.15. Structure of a polyethoxylated carboxylate. The -R group represents an alkyl group and M is a cation. The subscript n denotes the degree of ethoxylation.

## Amphoteric Detergents

Amphoteric detergents are an important class of detergents, which are milder to the skin in terms of TEWL of the scalp and moisture retention. They have been used in special detangling 2 in 1 shampoos since the mid-1970s. The use of amphoteric detergents became novel when a special cationic polymer, based upon a cellulose moiety, was formulated with amphoteric detergents and crypto anionic detergents as a detangling shampoo (Gerstein, 1976, p. 1).

The apparent incompatibility of cationic polymers and anionic detergents was overcome by using amphoteric detergents along with crypto anionic detergents. This was a technology breakthrough, where the hair was able to be cleansed and conditioned at the same time. These shampoos overconditioned Type 1 and Type 2 straight Caucasian hair, but they became very popular for African-descent haircare because of the detangling properties they conferred to wavy and curly/coily Type 3 and Type 4 hair, which tangles the most and is less prone to over-conditioning (Khalil & Syed, 1980, p. 1).

Amphoteric detergents are detergents that carry both a positive and a negative charge. They act as a positively charged species like conditioners below a pH of 6 and as cleansing anionic detergents at alkaline pH of 8 and 9. The most commonly used classes of amphoteric detergents are acetates, propionates, glycinates, amino propionates, betaines, and hydroxysultaines. The structures of these classes are shown in the following sections.

### Class 1A: Amphoteric Acetates and Propionates

Amphoacetate is a commonly used detergent, but it contains very high levels of sodium chloride (1-12%), which interfere with the formation of a complex between cationic polymers and anionic detergents. The cationic-amphoteric-anionic complex is less stable and coats the hair with unwanted polymeric residue. The structure of disodium cocoamphodiacetate is shown in **Figure 5.16**.

Amphopropionate is also a commonly used detergent; it is further treated to remove most of the sodium chloride. The complex formed between amphopropionate, cationic polymer, and anionic detergent is more stable. This complex does not coat the hair with unwanted polymeric residue. The structure of disodium cocoamphodipropionate is shown in

**Figure 5.17.**

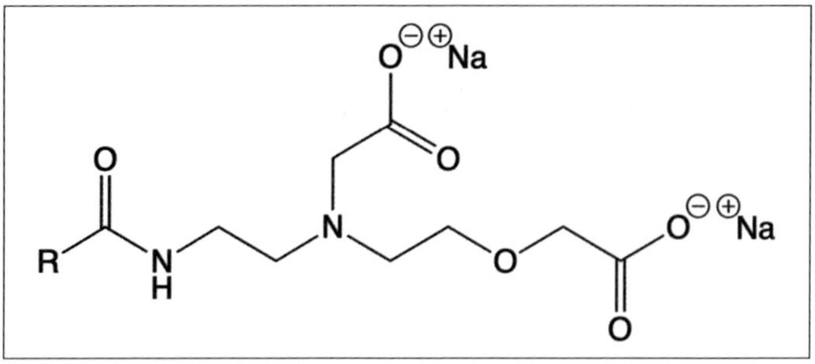

Figure 5.16. Structure of disodium cocoamphodiacetate. The -R group represents mixed coconut acid moieties.

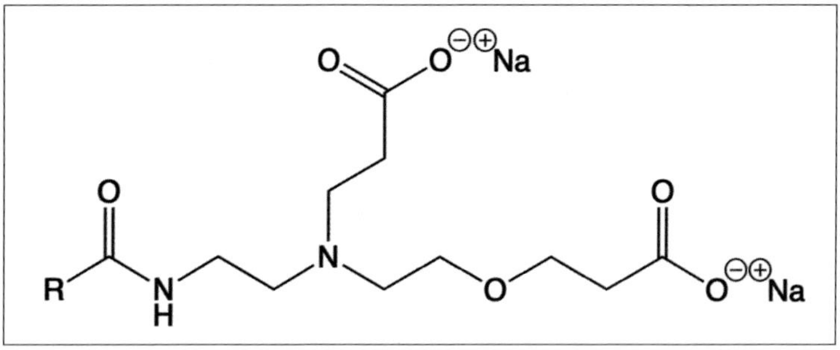

Figure 5.17. Structure of disodium cocoamphodipropionate. The -R group represents mixed coconut acid moieties.

When disodium cocoamphodipropionate was patch-tested on a human forearm against a control, there was a significant difference in the TEWL values of the control's untreated skin against disodium cocoamphodipropionate at $p < .05$ (Syed et al., 2008, p. 34). Although this compound is considered gentle to the skin, it still disrupts the stratum corneum, when compared to untreated skin.

For a premium Type 4 hair and scalp shampoo, normally a high level of amphoteric detergent such as sodium cocoamphoacetate or disodium cocoamphodipropionate is included in the formulation with a small amount of an anionic detergent such as disodium alkyl sulfosuccinate and sodium cocoyl isethionate to boost foaming. These combinations of detergents in a shampoo are mild and do not dry out the hair and scalp.

### Class 1B: Betaines

These compounds are zwitterions, carrying both a positive and negative charge. Quite a few betaines are used in formulating shampoos; the most commonly used betaine is cocamidopropyl betaine (CAPB). The structure of this compound is shown in **Figure 5.18**.

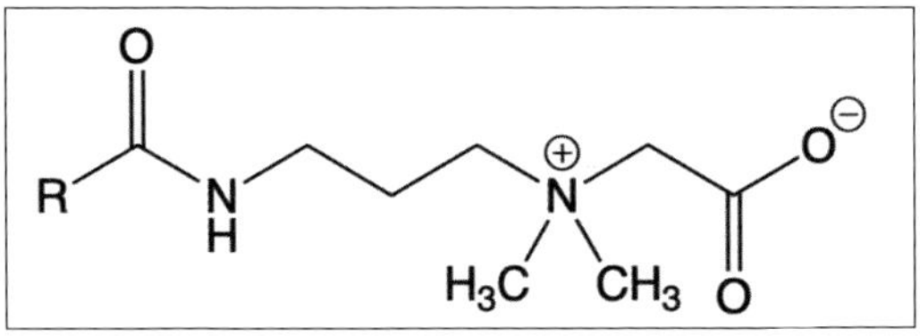

**Figure 5.18.** Structure of cocamidopropyl betaine. The -RCO group represents fatty acids derived from coconut oil.

When cocamidopropyl betaine (CAPB) was patch-tested on a human forearm against a control, there was no significant difference in the TEWL values of the control's untreated skin against CAPB, at $p = .343$, which is $> .05$ (Syed et al., 2008, p. 37).

Hydroxysultaines, also called sulfobetaines, are gentle to the skin like cocamidopropyl betaine. The structure of two common hydroxysultaines, lauryl hydroxysultaine and cocamidopropyl hydroxysultaine, are shown in **Figures 5.19** and **5.20** respectively.

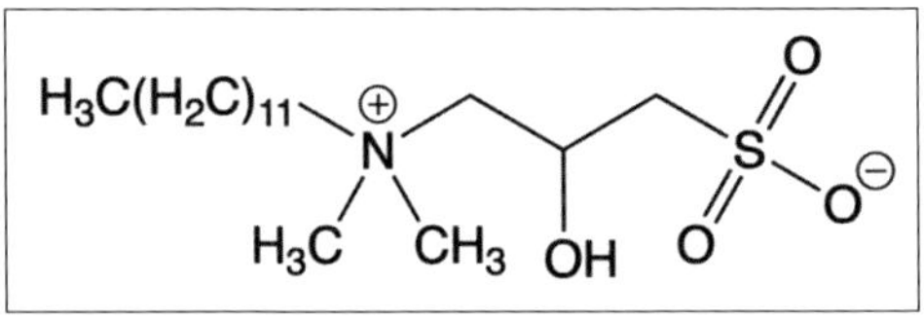

**Figure 5.19.** Structure of lauryl hydroxysultaine.

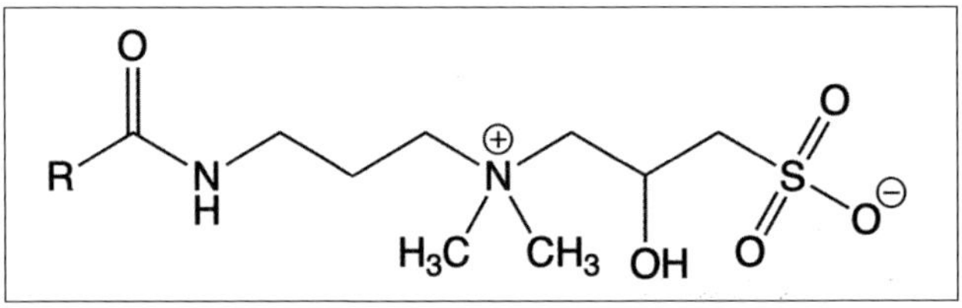

**Figure 5.20.** Structure of cocamidopropyl hydroxysultaine. The -RCO group represents fatty acids derived from coconut oil.

Of the two hydroxysultaines, lauryl hydoxysultaine produces higher viscosity than cocamidopropyl hydroxysultaine when combined with anionic or amphoteric detergents.

## Nonionic Detergents

The most commonly used detergents in this class are alkyl glucosides, which are condensation products of natural fatty alcohols and natural glucose. The general structure of an alkyl glucoside is shown in **Figure 5.21**, where -R represents an alkyl group from anywhere between 2 to 22 carbons in length and the subscript n refers to the degree of polymerization of the glucose monomer. For example, a degree of polymerization of 2 means di-glucose, maltose. Regardless of the degree of polymerization, these detergents are named "glucosides."

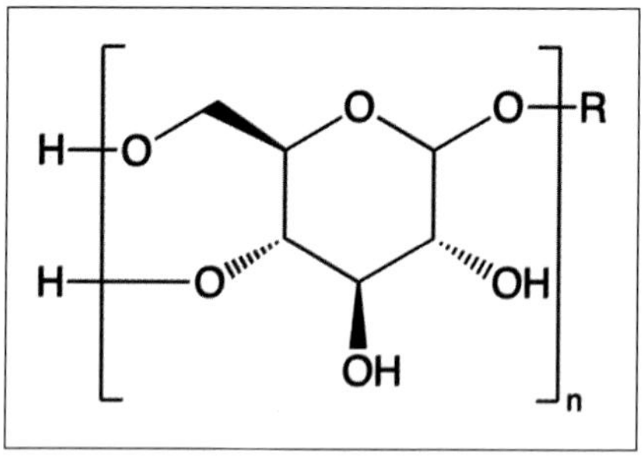

Figure 5.21. Structure of an alkyl glucoside where -R represents an alkyl group from anywhere between 2 to 22 carbons in length. The subscript n refers to the degree of polymerization of the glucose monomer. Regardless of the degree of polymerization, these ingredients are named "glucosides".

They are moderate in their foaming ability and biodegradable, but shampoos containing them are difficult to thicken. These detergents are becoming more popular nowadays because of the demand for natural products. The most popular glucosides are decyl glucoside, coco glucoside, and lauryl glucoside, among others.

## Cationic Surfactants

Cationic surfactants are quaternary ammonium compounds, which carry a positively charged moiety that can attach itself to the negatively charged sites of hair fibers. The general structure of a cationic surfactant is shown in **Figure 5.22**.

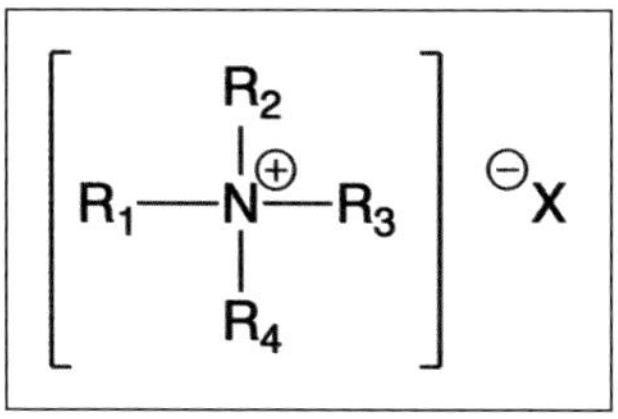

**Figure 5.22.** Structure of a quaternary ammonium compound, where $R_1$, $R_2$, $R_3$, and $R_4$ represent alkyl or aryl groups and X is an anion such as, but not limited to, a halide or sulfate.

The substituted nitrogen part of the molecule acts as a cation, that is, positively charged. Quaternary ammonium compounds are poor foaming agents, but they act as surfactants, and some of them could be employed as cleansing agents. An example of a quaternary ammonium compound used for cleansing hair is cetrimonium chloride (cetyl trimethyl ammonium chloride), but it is a poor foamer, as compared to alkyl sulfates, alkyl ether sulfates, and amphoteric detergents. The structure of cetrimonium chloride is shown in **Figure 5.23**.

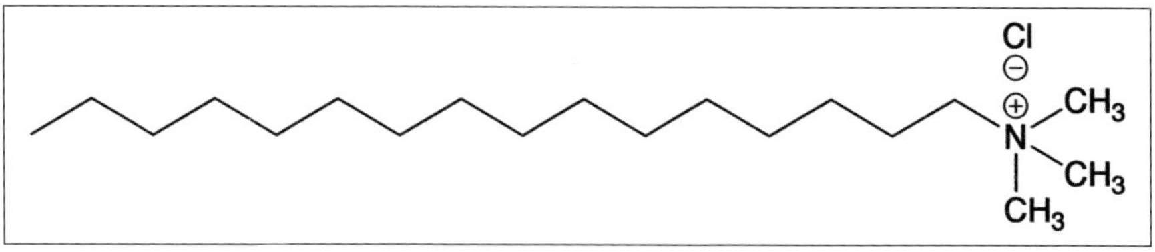

**Figure 5.23.** Structure of cetrimonium chloride, which includes one cetyl group and three methyl groups attached to the quaternary nitrogen. The counteranion is chloride.

Another group of quaternary compounds that act as cleansers are amine oxides. The general structure of an amine oxide (**Figure 5.24a**), as well as specific examples of two common amine oxides are shown in **Figure 5.24**.

Amine oxides foam relatively well, and cleanse and condition the hair simultaneously. Both cetrimonium chloride and coamidopropylamine

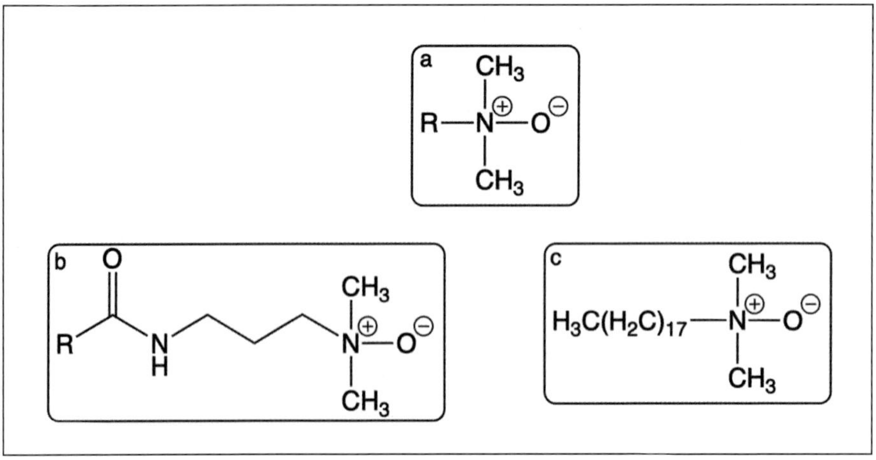

**Figure 5.24.** (a) General structure of an alkyl amine oxide where -R represents an alkyl or alkylamido group. (b) Structure of cocamidopropylamine oxide where -R represents fatty acids derived from coconut oil. (c) Structure of stearamine oxide.

oxide (see **Figure 5.24b** for structure) can be used in low-foaming cleansing conditioners, especially suitable for curly and coily hair types where cleansing products are not required to foam highly. Cocamidopropylamine oxide is readily biodegradable and is a better choice in formulations with amine oxides (Garcia, Campos, Ribosa, 2007, p. 1578).

Amine oxides help to stabilize foam and also to build viscosity of shampoos. You may recognize various amine oxides in your products in the ingredient listing as cocamidopropylamine oxide, soyamidopropylamine oxide, tallowamidopropylamine oxide, cocamine oxide, stearamine oxide (see **Figure 5.24c** for structure), oleamine oxide, and tallowamine oxide.

A discussion of quaternary ammonium compounds as hair conditioners is presented in greater detail in the next chapter.

## Natural Detergents

Saponins are present in natural ingredients such as in soap nuts, which are also known as *Sapindus mukorossi,* with the common name of reetha. It is a species of tree in the family of Sapindaceae. Reetha or Areetha is available in Pakistan and India. Reetha contains saponins, which are known for their moderate foam and cleansing properties. Reetha extract at

13.25% has a pH of 6.5; it foams well but not like sodium lauryl or laureth sulfate. The addition of reasonable amounts of sulfate-free detergent can produce desirable foam, if needed. Reetha extract is also very difficult to thicken; formulating chemists can thicken reetha extract with polymers such as xanthan gum to achieve desired viscosity.

Another natural plant called shikakai, with the Latin name Acacia Concinna, is a native shrub of Asia, especially of central and south India and southern Punjab in Pakistan. The hydrolyzed plant yields lupeol, spinasterol, acacic acid, lactone, and natural sugars such as glucose, arabinose, and rhamnose. It also contains oxalic acid, tartaric acid, citric acid, succinic acid, ascorbic acid, and alkaloids. The pH of the extract of shikakai is around 6.5. The comparison of foam produced from reetha, shikakai, and sodium lauryl sulfate solutions is shown in **Figure 5.25**. As expected, the sodium lauryl sulfate solutions (5.0% and 13.25% active) produced the most foam, followed by reetha extract, while shikakai did not produce appreciable foam. Thus, reetha extract is able to cleanse hair well and produce foam, although not as well as sodium lauryl sulfate.

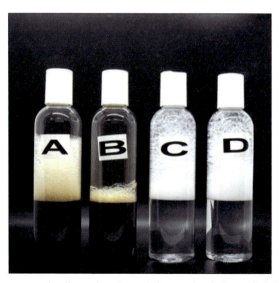

Figure 5.25. Foam production of various detergent solutions. Solution A is 13.25% aqueous extract of reetha. Solution B is 13.25% aqueous extract of shikakai. Solution C is 5.0% active, aqueous sodium lauryl sulfate. Solution D is 13.25% active, aqueous sodium lauryl sulfate. Each solution was inverted 20 times to produce foam.

## Hair & Scalp Prior to Shampooing

The area of the human scalp is roughly 100–108 square inches (650–700 square centimeters) with 100,000 to 150,000 hairs covering the scalp (Beauquey, 2005, p. 93). Similarly, the area of the hair on the human head will vary depending on the length of the hair. A rough estimate of the area of hair surface is 54–215 square feet, or 5–20 square meters (p. 93). This area would be the equivalent to a 14 x 14 foot room. Thus, 1 to 2 fluid ounces of a shampoo has to cleanse this large surface area of the hair and scalp in two to three minutes of application and contact time.

In the shampooing process, the nature of the hair surface must be evaluated with respect to chemical damage and styling-product buildup, and the condition of the scalp must be evaluated as well, as all of these factors play an important role in proper and healthy cleansing. Normally, hair picks up soil from environmental contaminants such as pollution and dust made of clay that contains iron oxide (Wong, 1997, p. 34). Additionally, the hair's surface may be loaded with hair spray or hair gel and petrolatum-based leave-on products. Conditions of the scalp vary significantly from consumer to consumer with respect to secretion of sebum from the sebaceous glands and the cell turnover as debris from scalp desquamation, which may also contain proteins and organic/mineral components as part of sweat. The African-descent scalp does not secrete as much sebum as the Caucasian scalp and tends to be drier. Therefore, African-descent consumers tend to shampoo their hair and scalp once per week or once every two weeks, as compared to the daily shampooing ritual of Caucasians. In the absence of daily shampooing, African-descent hair and scalp collect significant quantities of debris over two weeks. The African-descent scalp also collects plenty of microorganisms (bacteria, fungi, etc.) during this gap between shampoo treatments. Some of the types of microorganisms on the African-descent scalp surface are *Citrobacter, Staphylococcus aureus,* and *Malassezia species* fungus (Syed, 2008, p. 2). The secreted debris, which is a mixture of pollutants from the environment, topical leave-on products, cell turnover from the scalp, sebum from sebaceous glands, and sweat from sweat glands is sticky in nature and not easy to remove. It was common in African-descent salons until the mid-1990s to scrape the surface of the customer's scalp upon arrival, before shampooing. It sometimes took 45 to 50 minutes for this process. After scraping the scalp with a rattail comb, hair stylists proceeded to apply alcoholic anti-bacterial products to disinfect the scalp, followed by shampooing. This whole process was very painful for consumers, but they still opted for this service in order to attain a clean scalp. This state of affairs gave birth to a new hair care regimen based on mild shampoos containing anti-bacterial and anti-fungal shampoos and conditioners, typically known as "Dry and Itchy" shampoo, and "Dry & Itchy" Conditioner, and a topical "Dry & Itchy" leave-in product that replaced this painful archaic process. To date, this regimen is a leading treatment in African-descent salons for dry and itchy scalp, which removes bacteria and fungus from the scalp during the process. The effects of the fungus may also play a role in scalp-related diseases and loss of hair.

## The Physics of Hair & Scalp Cleansing

The detergents in shampoos weaken the physiochemical bonds between the sticky debris and the surface of the hair and scalp, thereby transferring the debris to the aqueous medium of the shampoo. Upon rinsing with water, almost 99.5% of the debris leaves the surface of the hair and scalp and becomes part of the rinse water. It is important to know that surfactants are molecules with two parts: one part is lipophilic (oil loving), and the other part is hydrophilic (water loving). For example, the geometric shape of an anionic detergent is shown in **Figure 5.26**. Initially the lipophilic part of the detergent mixes with the oily debris on the surface of the hair and scalp. Then, the hydrophilic part of the detergent makes the detergent and the sticky debris miscible with water, which allows the rinsing of all surface debris. This process is responsible for the effective cleansing of the hair and scalp.

A schematic of cleansing of debris from the surface of the hair and scalp by the shampoo is shown in **Figure 5.27**.

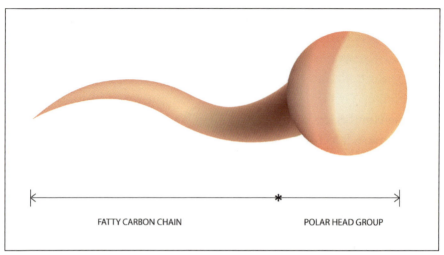

**Figure 5.26.** Schematic of the geometry and shape of an anionic detergent.

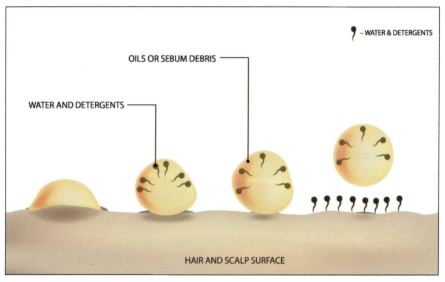

**Figure 5.27.** Schematic of oil and sebum removal (cleansing) from the surface of the hair and scalp.

## The Effect of Detergents on the Hair

Detergents can affect hair and skin with respect to pH, moisture content, transepidermal water loss, cuticle hair proteins, the CMC of the cuticle layers, 18-MEA (F layer) of the cuticle layers, and fiber elasticity.

**pH.** The detergents in the shampoo can alter the pH of the hair and scalp, particularly detergents with alkaline pH. This increase in pH is not a desirable attribute, as the hair and scalp are healthiest in the average pH range of 5.0-5.8 (Schmid-Wendtner & Korting, 2007, p. 15). An acidic pH offers favorable conditions for apathogenic resident flora and unfavorable conditions for pathogenic flora; for example, *Staphylococcus aureus* is negatively affected at pH 5.5 of the scalp, thus reducing the chances of inflammatory skin lesions in acne-prone individuals. Similarly, high TEWL values are related to high pH, low hydration, and reduced skin lipids (p. 78). This is one of the reasons that alkaline shampoos, soap bars, and shampoos based on soaps (sodium stearate or potassium stearate) are not good for the hair and scalp, becoming relatively obsolete in the cosmetics industry. However, recently certified organic shampoos that contain soaps have become popular. These types of shampoos are not desirable because they increase the pH of the hair and scalp, decrease hair and scalp moisture, and increase scalp TEWL.

**Moisture content and surface lipids of the hair and scalp.** It is important to select a shampoo formulation that contains optimum concentrations of mild detergents, so that the TEWL, moisture, and surface lipids of the scalp and hair are not altered. For example, sodium lauryl sulfate, ammonium lauryl sulfate, and alpha olefin sulfonates will increase TEWL, reducing the moisture, and hence drying the scalp, especially in the case of African-descent scalp that is inherently dry to begin with. Determination of hair moisture through a microwave resonance technique indicated that hair also loses moisture when treated with sodium lauryl sulfate and ammonium lauryl sulfate (Syed et al., 2008, p. 33). The new trend among consumers with curly hair is to use low-foaming shampoos to keep the moisture of the hair and scalp intact along with its surface lipids. Over the last decade, a new category of hair and scalp cleansers has emerged, known as Co-Wash cleansers. These cleansers do not contain shampoo-type anionic detergents but contain quaternary compounds that foam less in order to preserve the moisture, TEWL, and surface lipids of the hair and scalp. The Co-Wash cleansers are very popular among consumers with Type 3 and Type 4 wavy, curly, and coily hair.

**Loss of cuticle proteins during shampooing and wet combing.** During the cleansing process, the cuticles swell to some degree in wet conditions, and some of these cuticles detach from the hair shaft during shampooing and wet-combing and rinse away with water (Sandhu et al., 1995, p. 39). Greater quantities of harsh detergents in shampoos are also responsible for the shedding of small amounts of the cuticles and the cell membrane complex (CMC) between the cuticle-cuticle layer of the innermost cuticle layer and the outermost cortical layer. Shedding of the cuticles is equated with loss of hair protein and a small but significant loss of hair elasticity.

The Sandhu et al. (1995) study collected the chipped-away cuticles after shampoo treatment and wet-combing (p. 50). These cuticles were hydrolyzed and analyzed for their protein content. The researchers demonstrated that significant quantities of protein from the cuticles were lost during the shampooing process. It was also shown that hair tresses treated with non-conditioning shampoos were losing more hair proteins during wet-combing than those treated with detangling shampoos. The loss of cuticles increased hair porosity and decreased hair elasticity. Just a single shampoo treatment using a shampoo that contained a harsh detergent reduced hair elasticity significantly.

It is also believed that while cleansing the hair during repeated shampoo treatments, the lipids present on the upper surface of the hair, that are covalently attached to cystine in the cuticles, such as 18-MEA, may unravel, slightly dissolve in harsh detergents, and wash away upon rinsing the hair, thus rendering the hair surface somewhat porous and dull. The use of conditioners helps in replenishing these lost lipids, which are not covalently bonded to cystine of the cuticles. This lipid replenishment is temporary; it lasts from one treatment to the next.

## The Effect of Detergents on the Skin

Many shampoos in the marketplace use approximately 10-15% active concentration of detergents to cleanse the hair effectively. Therefore, a study was conducted by Syed et al. (2008), using various detergents, each with a 15.0% concentration. The skin patch test was applied to the forearm with a closed chamber technique, and each detergent was left on the arm for 4 hours. The patch was removed, the forearm was rinsed with water, and the arm was allowed to rest for 1 hour. Bioengineering techniques were utilized to measure skin moisture, skin TEWL, skin pH, and skin erythema. Skin erythema was evaluated with a spectrophotometric erythema meter, as well as visually. The visual observations for skin irritation were not discriminating.

After removing the patch, TEWL readings were taken for 14 different detergents, and the analysis of variance (ANOVA) was conducted on the resultant data using a Tukey B test. The results indicated that sodium lauryl sulfate, ammonium lauryl sulfate, sodium $C_{12-14}$ olefin sulfonate, and sodium lauroyl sarcosinate increased TEWL significantly, at $p < .05$ (Syed et al., 2008, p. 39). It was also observed that TEWL values corresponding to sodium laureth sulfate were not significantly greater than TEWL of untreated skin, at $p = .110$. The marketing campaign of "sulfate-free" shampoos may have validity, but scientific results have shown that sodium laureth sulfate and ammonium laureth sulfate from the class of sulfated detergents were mild to the skin with respect to their effect on the stratum corneum.

It was also found that most of the detergents at 15.0% concentration affected the TEWL of the skin significantly. The TEWL recovery of the skin took a few days in most cases. The important findings of the study were that most detergents will dry out the skin initially and that it takes longer than 48 hours for the skin to recover its lost moisture. In the case of a few detergents such as cocamidopropyl betaine, cocamidopropyl hydroxysultaine, and sodium cocoyl isethionate, the skin recovered its TEWL within 48 hours ($p < .05$). Therefore, these three detergents were considered relatively gentle (Syed et al., 2008, pp. 37, 40).

## Mitigating Shampoo Damage

When shampoo is applied to wet hair, it is customary to manipulate the hair and scalp in order to create sufficient sudsing, or lather. This manipulation ends up detaching some of the cuticles from the surface of the hair, and hair fibers also lose some of the cuticle CMC (cuticle glue).

This loss of hair cuticles and CMC is responsible for a significant reduction of hair elasticity. In addition, the stratum corneum, or the TEWL value of the scalp, is altered, and it may take from 48 hours to 1 week for the stratum corneum of the skin to recover and return to its original state.

The hair becomes difficult to comb in both the wet and dry states after shampoo treatment. Type 4 hair was found to be 23 times more difficult to comb, thus rendering combing as a painful process in which the scalp experiences a great deal of pulling force. Individuals of Type 4 hair with a tender scalp may even cry due to pain during combing. If the scalp has a condition of psoriasis, the inflammation of the scalp increases due to harsh shampoo detergents that are irritating and drying.

In order to mitigate shampooing damage, one must select a shampoo composed of mild detergents along with moisturizing and detangling ingredients such as cationic polymers. When included in detangling shampoos, these cationic polymers aid in detangling Types 3 and 4 hair effectively. They also help reduce friction created by hair and scalp manipulation during the shampooing process. When gentle detergents are used, they reduce the loss of moisture, maintain the stratum corneum, preserve hair elasticity, and reduce shedding of cuticles and their CMC from the surface of the hair. After shampooing, an application of well-formulated conditioners will help reduce much of the damage caused by the shampooing process.

The protection of curly/coily Types 3 and 4 hair, against shampoo damage is very important because of the difficulty of combing this type of hair. Shampoos for curly and coily hair are formulated with the following features in mind: The base of the shampoo contains detergents that are very gentle to the hair and scalp with a view toward preserving the scalp's stratum corneum and its moisture, along with the moisture of the hair. The base is tested on the hair and scalp to ensure that hair moisture, the pH of the hair and scalp, and the TEWL of the scalp are preserved. Also, the scalp is tested for any irritation or inflammation from the chosen detergents. Upon successfully choosing the detergents, other additives are included in the formulation. Conditioning additives such as cationic polymers are added to impart detangling properties to the hair. This feature of the shampoo is crucial for Type 3 and Type 4 hair.

Shampooing damage is also reduced with the use of conditioners that will replenish hair and scalp moisture, reduce TEWL values of the scalp in order to repair the stratum corneum, neutralize any detergents still present on the surface of the hair, balance the pH of the hair and scalp, and fortify the CMC of the cuticles with the use of lipids such as ceramides, phytosphingosines, and cholesterol.

New products are developed through a multidisciplinary approach where not only chemists but scientists with various backgrounds take part in the process. For example, formulation chemists, physicists, biotechnologists, hairstylists, chemical engineers, dermatologists, analytical chemists, quality assurance scientists, marketing specialists, and consultants/contract laboratories work together to help develop a new product. This multidisciplinary approach helps to develop new world-class products. Therefore, it is important to look at the most important steps in the process of developing new products in a research and development (R&D) laboratory.

## The Product Development Process

The six major steps involved in the process of developing a new product are as follows:

1. Product development request
2. Inputs
3. Prototype development
4. Independent outside testing of the prototype
5. Test market
6. National launch

A flow chart of the product development process is shown in **Figure 5.28**.

### Step 1 – Product Development Request

This step reviews consumer needs, economic viability of the product, and important parameters that need to be considered while

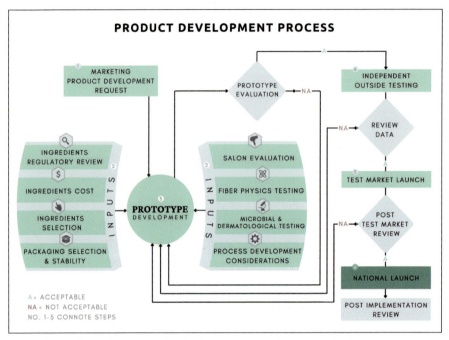

Figure 5.28. Flow-diagram of a six-step process of new product development.

developing the product. The instructions or inputs are provided to R&D for developing the product and contain such information as perceived product characteristics, regulatory review of the inputs regarding safety of ingredients, ingredient costs, compatibility of the product with packaging components, appropriateness of product dispensing from the packaging components, competitive pricing versus prototype costs and price, and profitability of the new product. A sample of a product development request form or PDR is shown in Exhibit A.

### Step 2 – Inputs

The marketing department of an organization researches the attributes of the new product, its functional elements, its market prospect or consumer demand, the cost of the ingredients, type of packaging components, and the final price for consumers.

Formulating chemists gather appropriate ingredients, and information regarding the cost, safety, consumer acceptance, and the regulatory status of these ingredients.

### Step 3 – Prototype Development

The approved and selected ingredients are converted into a prototype, and the protype is initially tested on hair tresses for its performance and product specifications in a quality assurance laboratory. If the results are encouraging, the prototype is submitted to a company hair salon for testing on humans. The prototype is tested on humans using a half-head technique where the prototype is tested against a standard product. The salon test results are evaluated, appropriate changes are made in the prototype, and the prototype is retested in the hair salon. The results of the salon retest are evaluated, and feedback is given to the formulating chemist.

After the preliminary evaluation of the prototype, it is submitted to various laboratories such as a fiber physics laboratory, a dermatology laboratory, and a microbiology laboratory. The needed claims are evaluated in these laboratories. For example, for a new shampoo prototype, the fiber physics laboratory can test for ease of wet combing, ease of dry combing, moisturization, increase or decrease in hair elasticity, increase or decrease in the static charge during dry combing, decrease of friction between hair fibers during combing, and hair surface damage after shampooing.

A dermatology laboratory uses bioengineering techniques to measure the moisture of the scalp before and after treatment with the shampoo, the impact of the shampoo on the stratum corneum of the scalp (TEWL), pH of the scalp, any erythema or irritation of the scalp, and surface examination of the scalp.

An analytical chemistry laboratory determines the loss of cuticles in the form of proteins from the surface of the hair during shampooing. Other relevant analytical chemistry tests are also conducted.

Quality assurance and quality control laboratories test the compatibility of the prototype with the packaging components of the prototype and the stability of the active ingredients, if present, in the prototype such as zinc pyrithione as an antidandruff ingredient. If performance is dissatisfactory in any of the tests in various laboratories, the prototype is improved in the formulation laboratory and re-evaluation is conducted in each of the laboratories once more. When the prototype passes all tests in all of the laboratories, the prototype is ready for the next step.

## Step 4 – Independent Outside Testing

Independent outside testing is conducted using various techniques. One of the ways is the so-called focus group test, which is based on blind testing of the prototype with consumers or hairstylists. The test is normally conducted by an independent market research specialist. Data are collected by the specialist, and an independent report is issued. Another market test is based on survey research, where the market research specialists provide the sample of the prototype and the survey questionnaire to hundreds of consumers, while keeping the identity of the organization confidential. The consumers use the product according to the directions provided and return the questionnaire after use with their comments, which are tabulated by the market research specialists, and product acceptance is gauged. If consumer acceptance is high and consumers show high purchase intent, the prototype is, then, sent for a test market launch.

## Step 5 – Test Market Launch

This step is sometimes bypassed by smaller organizations due to a lack of resources or because of an urgency to introduce the product to gain market share or to cope with competitive pressures. Recently, smaller brands have started introducing their prototypes to loyal customers via social media. The new product is launched virtually and fans are informed about the launch via social media. Fans of the brand buy the product directly from the company, use it, and then review the product on various social media platforms. This consumer feedback helps the brand to review the product performance and make decisions regarding go or nogo of a national launch.

## Step 6 – National Launch

New products are introduced to consumers through national distribution organizations that have physical stores throughout the United States. Over the last two decades, products have also been introduced to consumers through online sales organizations such as Amazon. A national launch is expensive, and product performance, price, and promotions all play important roles in the success of the launch. If the launch is successful, the dividends are appreciable, but if the launch is not successful, the losses are substantial as well. The long-term success of a brand and its organization depend upon successful launches. Therefore, the professionals involved in the introduction of new products must understand the factors involved in the success of new products.

## Types of Shampoos

A shampoo should cleanse the hair and scalp thoroughly, while producing adequate rich lather in order to remove excess sebum and buildup of styling products from the hair. However, the detergents used in the shampoo should be gentle to the hair and nonirritating to the scalp, and the shampoo should be able to normalize the pH of hair and scalp to between 5.0-5.8 in order to provide resistance to unwanted bacteria and support a positive scalp environment for hair growth. The shampoo should be non-damaging and moisturizing to the hair and scalp, and it should not disturb the stratum corneum. The shampoo should also rinse easily, and leave the hair in a easy to comb state, feeling light, having a lot of body and shine, and with a lasting style (Beauquey, 2005, p. 84).

Formulating shampoos for curly hair types can be challenging because of the needs and conditions of curly/coily hair and scalp. Just to review: Curly/coily hair is 23 times more difficult to comb in the wet state and 32 times more difficult to comb in the dry state (Syed, et al., 2022, p.49). Curly/coily hair is more fragile with 33% less elasticity than straight hair (p. 50). Curly/coily hair has 30% less moisture than straight hair, and the scalp of African-descent individuals displays 20% less moisture and 28% higher TEWL values. Thus, the stratum corneum of the African-descent scalp is significantly weaker than that of Caucasian scalp (p. 50).

Since wet African-descent hair is very different in its attributes, the shampoos for hair and scalp should have the following properties: The shampoo should cleanse hair and scalp gently and impart detangling properties during wet and dry combing of the hair in order to eliminate the combing and brushing damage. It should be moisturizing to hair and scalp with an unaltered stratum corneum. The pH of the hair and scalp should be normalized between 5.0 and 5.8, perhaps by using gentle organic acids, in order to create favorable conditions for an apathogenic resident flora, thus reducing the chances of scalp inflammation. Hair-strengthening ingredients should also be added in order to reduce hair fragility and increase hair elasticity. Finally, the shampoo should impart the rest of the properties such as ease of rinsing from hair, hair softness, ease of styling, hair bounciness, antistatic condition, and hair sheen.

This is a long list of attributes that a shampoo formulation must address, and it is not easy to attain all of these attributes in a single shampoo formulation. That is why shampoos are classified into many different categories such as cleansing/clarifying shampoos, detangling shampoos, antidandruff shampoos, shampoos for damaged hair, moisturizing shampoos, shampoos for color-treated hair, dry powder shampoos, and coloring shampoos. Each category is formulated according to the desired attributes for a targeted group of consumers.

Currently, many types of shampoos are marketed to consumers. But does it make sense to market different types of shampoos to consumers? The answer to this question is a resounding yes. The reason behind this answer is the great variation in hair textures, varying scalp, and varying needs of consumers who are depending on proper conditioning of their hair and scalp. Also, the build-up of leave-on products dictates the type of shampoo to be used on a specific individual's hair and scalp. The various types of shampoos currently marketed for textured hair are as follows:

- Cleansing and Clarifying Shampoo
- Co-Wash Cleansers
- Detangling/Conditioning Shampoo
- Moisturizing Shampoo
- Anti-dandruff Shampoo
- Shampoo for Damaged Hair
- Shampoo for Color-Treated Hair
- Shampoo for Thinning and Falling Hair

- Baby Shampoo
- Dry Powder Shampoo
- Coloring Shampoos

**Cleansing and clarifying shampoos.** Cleansing and clarifying shampoos are commonly used to cleanse the hair and scalp and remove heavy buildup of leave-on styling products such as styling gels, holding sprays, pomades made of petrolatum, waxes from styling products, and mineral oils. Current cleansing/clarifying shampoos usually contain sodium lauryl sulfate or ammonium lauryl sulfate or sodium olefin sulfonate or a combination of these detergents at 10-15% active concentrations. These shampoos usually disturb the moisture balance of the hair and scalp and damage the stratum corneum of the scalp. Over the last decade, a new trend of "sulfate-free" shampoos has become popular where lauryl/laureth sulfates are replaced with gentler detergents such as nonsulfated sulfosuccinates, amphoteric detergents, acyl isethionates, alkyl glucosides, and amino acid-derived detergents, to name a few. While formulating sulfate-free shampoos, the types and concentrations of detergents need to be selected with care to arrive at a mild shampoo formula that is less drying to hair and scalp and non-disturbing to the stratum corneum.

The development of the formulation should be based on a modular approach. The various modules of a shampoo formulation are as follows:

- Water is the carrier of all ingredients. Water quality should be tested for conductivity, pH, total organic content, and for the absence of bacteria.
- Detergents should be selected based upon their gentleness to the hair and scalp in terms of moisture and TEWL.
- The pH of the shampoo system must be in the range of 5.0-5.8 to provide optimum pH for skin and hair against pathogenic flora.
- Foam boosters such as alkanolamides should be added at a minimum level, just to achieve the desired foaming. Consumers are no longer looking for high-foaming shampoos.

- Fragrance should be selected based upon its safety profile and the absence of endocrine disruptors.
- The shampoo should produce flash foam when applied to wet hair.
- The shampoo should not be too thick, otherwise it will not produce flash foam.
- The shampoo should rinse out easily.

The new product development steps are listed in the new product development flow chart of Figure 5.28. They should be followed in order to optimize the development of a quality product with shorter development time. The safety and regulatory profile of all ingredients should be reviewed before proceeding to formulation work. The amount of detergent and other relevant ingredients must be optimized to meet the desired attributes of the product. If detergents are used at higher concentration than needed, they may strip the moisture from the hair and scalp and may damage the stratum corneum. The formula should be tested in a hair salon for all attributes such as foam, removal of all debris from the hair and scalp, perceived moisture of the hair and scalp, rinsability, shine, and any other required attributes in the marketing profile. During salon testing, the scalp moisture and TEWL of the salon patrons' scalp must be measured and brought to the desired level using bioengineering techniques in a dermatology laboratory. Upon successful salon testing and dermatological testing, the scalp should have proper moisture content and an undisturbed stratum corneum. A fiber physics laboratory should also verify the moisture content of the hair. If the dermatological testing does not yield positive results, the quantities of detergent and other relevant ingredients should be readjusted to achieve favorable results in terms of moisture and TEWL of the scalp. If the hair and scalp gain moisture and the scalp TEWL decreases, then the formula should be tested in a claims substantiation laboratory for appropriate marketing claims. This process is repeated until all goals are achieved.

The formula should also be tested for preservation against microbial growth, stability at elevated temperatures, and product-packaging stability.

The regulatory and safety parameters should be reviewed once more before testing the prototype in a market test for consumer acceptance. If the shampoo formula passes all criteria set forth in the marketing profile, then the product should be introduced to the marketplace.

**Co-wash cleansing conditioners.** As one of the most recent phenomena in the marketplace, this category of cleansers satisfies the new demands of consumers who possess Type 3 and Type 4 wavy, curly, or coily hair. Generally, consumers with Type 4 hair have a dry scalp, and washing the hair becomes quite cumbersome on a daily or an every-three-day basis. It is a well-known fact that 90% of consumers with Type 4 (African-descent) hair shampoo their hair every one to two weeks (Lewallen et al., 2015, p. 219). If a cleansing shampoo consisting of anionic detergents is used, the hair becomes very raspy and is very difficult to comb. Also, the relatively dry hair and dry scalp of African-descent consumers loses more moisture and becomes even more dry by frequent cleansing. Therefore, these consumers cleanse their hair and scalp with cream conditioners that contain cationic/quaternary ammonium compounds as surface-active agents. The term *Co-Wash* means washing hair with conditioners. The surface-active compounds present in Co-Wash products are positively charged and condition the hair while providing a significant degree of cleansing. Although quaternary ammonium compounds are poor foamers, they have become acceptable to consumers with Type 3 and Type 4 hair. Co-Wash products provide sufficient cleansing for dry hair and a dry scalp ($\approx 96\%$), which does not make the hair and scalp feel stripped of moisture and natural oils. Co-Wash products have become very popular for Type 3 and Type 4 consumers in both the ethnic and general market. Consumers with Type 4 hair may use a co-wash every two weeks, whereas consumers with Type 2C and Type 3A hair may use a co-wash every week. Most of these consumers will use a shampoo every four weeks.

Because the category of co-wash cleansing conditioners is relatively new, no studies were found through a review of the literature with respect to comparing their cleansing power against shampoos. However, the Avlon Research Center conducted studies comparing the cleansing power of co-wash against a cleansing shampoo. In the study, untreated, clean, wavy hair tresses were used. Initial sebum values were measured at three sites on each tress using a sebum measuring device. Hair tresses were soiled by applying 0.5 ml of synthetic sebum and left on for 30 minutes. Sebum values were measured again at three sites on each tress. Each test product was applied to the tresses and left on for 1 minute. The hair tresses were rinsed with tap water for 3 minutes, and tresses were left to air dry. When the tresses were dry, sebum values were measured again at three sites on each tress. The following results were found and conclusions were made from the study:

- The "sulfate free" shampoo removed 99% of sebum.
- Similarly, the co-wash cleansing conditioner removed 96% of sebum.
- An independent *t* test showed that the "sulfate free" shampoo cleansed the hair significantly better than the co-wash cleansing conditioner (Syed & Mathew, 2017, p. 6). However, this difference was acceptable for Type 3 and Type 4 dry-scalp individuals.
- The advantages of the co-wash cleansing conditioner over the "sulfate free" shampoo were its superior moisturizing properties for dry Type 4 hair and associated dry scalp and its ability to cleanse without negatively altering the SC of the scalp.

**Detangling/conditioning shampoos.** Detangling/conditioning shampoos are usually popular among consumers who have wavy, curly, or coily hair, which is difficult to comb as compared to straight hair. Detangling shampoos formulated for Type 4 hair contain much higher concentrations of detangling cationic polymers such as polyquaternium-6, -7, and -10, and cationic guar gums. In addition, these shampoos are formulated with a mixture of gentler amphoteric, nonionic, and anionic detergents for foam boosting. The amphoteric and anionic detergents make a complex with the cationic polymer that is stable, easy to rinse, and foams well. The purpose of this amphoteric-anionic-cationic complex is to provide ease of wet and dry combing and to make the hair feel soft.

The pH is adjusted with organic acids such as citric acid between 5-5.8 to provide the most desirable pH environment for the scalp and hair. The detergents used are gentle to the hair and scalp and do not strip moisture from the hair; they also keep the stratum corneum of the scalp intact. The primary purpose of these shampoos is to help with combing ease of wavy/curly/coily hair in the wet and dry states, which clarifying shampoos do not provide.

Other additives are also included, according to marketing claims. For example, moisturizing ingredients are added to almost all shampoos in order to maintain the moisture balance of the hair and scalp. Hair-strengthening agents such as fruit extracts, hydrolyzed proteins, Royal Jelly, and ceramides are added in order to compensate for loss of elasticity of hair fibers during combing and brushing. Preservatives are added to increase the shelf life of the shampoos and guard against microbial growth. Fragrances are added to create pleasing sensory properties of the product during use. It is important to choose fragrances with human safety in mind. A fragrance may contain numerous aromatic compounds that could be endocrine disruptors (ECDs or EDs). Endocrine disruptors have been linked to carcinogenic activity in the human body, and it is imperative to spell out the safety standards to fragrance providers beforehand. It is now possible to screen fragrances for the presence of endocrine disruptors before their use.

**Anti-dandruff shampoos**. Anti-dandruff shampoos are formulated to remove dandruff flakes from the hair scalp during cleansing. The continuous use of these shampoos helps to manage scalp dandruff. If their use is discontinued, dandruff will reappear within six weeks. Active anti-dandruff ingredients are zinc pyrithione, selenium sulfide, ketoconazole, sulfur, salicylic acid, and other FDA/REACH-approved materials. It is also important to select detergents that are gentler in terms of the moisture profile of the hair and scalp. Additional moisturizing ingredients are added to the formula base. For wavy, curly, and coily hair (Types 3 and 4), detangling ingredients are included in the anti-dandruff shampoo as well.

**Moisturizing shampoos**. Moisturizing shampoos are formulated for dry or damaged hair and scalp; they normally contain gentler amphoteric detergents along with ingredients that are known to impart moisture to the hair and scalp. The moisture of the scalp is normally determined before and after treatment with the shampoo, using bioengineering techniques such as TEWL and corneometry. Detangling ingredients may also be added if the moisturizing shampoo is formulated for wavy and curly/coily hair (Types 3 and 4). Even in the case of wavy hair, detangling ingredients such as guar hydroxylpropyltrimonium chloride may be added to detangle the hair. Today, most shampoos contain moisturizing ingredients, and a separate moisturizing shampoo does not need to be formulated and marketed, unless required by marketing professionals.

**Shampoos for oily hair and scalp.** Shampoos for oily hair and scalp normally contain higher concentration of detergents such as sodium laureth sulfate. The active concentration of detergents may be between 12-15% for normal hair, whereas shampoos for oily hair may contain as much as 15-18% of these detergents. Also, addition of conditioning and detangling ingredients is avoided while formulating these types of shampoos. The degree of removal of oils from an oily hair and scalp may be determined by using desquamation techniques or sebum measurements with a sebumeter. Such shampoos are damaging to wavy or curly/coily hair. Their use must be avoided at all cost. These shampoos deplete the natural moisture of the hair and scalp, damage the stratum corneum of the scalp, remove more cuticles from the hair surface, and deplete the hair of proteins and cuticular CMC.

**Shampoos for volumizing hair.** Shampoos for volumizing hair can be formulated similar to shampoos for oily hair and scalp. The purpose of a volumizing shampoo is to increase hair volume of straight, fine, and thin hair by effectively removing oils and sebum from the hair, which consequently increases the volume of the hair. Volumizing polymers are also included in the formulation. These types of shampoos are not appropriate for wavy or curly/coily types of hair, as these hair types naturally have high hair volume. There are certain hair volumizing ingredients marketed by the suppliers of cosmetic raw materials that purport to increase the diameter of hair fibers, but the substantiation of increase in the diameter of hair fibers has not been validated by independent testing laboratories.

**Shampoos for thinning and falling hair.** Shampoos for thinning and falling hair should be based on active compounds that can stop thinning and shedding of hair. There are only two types of ingredients that work to stop shedding and thinning of hair. Shedding and thinning could be caused by telogen effluvium (more than 15% of hairs in the Telogen phase) and would require either medical treatments such as minoxidil-based shampoos or alternative treatments. In the alternative treatment, the shampoo contains a combination of phytosterols, saw palmetto extract, niacinamide, biotin, fruit extracts, caffeine, copper peptide, and antifungus ingredients.

Medical treatments need FDA approval, whereas alternative botanical treatments are readily marketable and may help in stopping or reducing hair shedding and thinning; yet, hair growth claims cannot be made. The minoxidil or alternative botanical ingredients are added in a base formula of a detangling shampoos composed of gentle detergents, cationic polymers, moisturizing ingredients, pH of 5-5.8, anti-fungal ingredients, gentle preservatives, and gentle fragrances (that do not contain endocrine disruptors). This type of shampoo category is relatively new to the market, and the proof of performance is somewhat questionable. This shampoo category creates the perception of hair growth indirectly, in order to avoid potential conflict with drug claims.

**Baby shampoos.** Specially formulated for use on baby or infant hair, baby shampoos claim to be very gentle to a baby's hair, scalp, and eyes. The detergents used are amphoteric or non-ionic in nature and have very low irritancy. Again, for babies with wavy or curly/coily hair, general market baby shampoos are not good enough because they make the hair difficult to comb. Therefore, baby shampoos for Types 3 and 4 hair should contain a small concentration of cationic polymer, a pH of 5-5.8, very gentle preservatives, and possibly no fragrance. Usually, baby shampoos are tested ophthalmologically on eyes of human subjects for a "no-tears" claim.

**Swimmers' shampoo.** Swimmers have a unique need besides merely cleansing their hair and scalp. During swimming, hair absorbs chlorine from the swimming pool water. The chlorine is used as a disinfectant for swimming pool water in order to inhibit bacterial growth. The negative consequence of this chlorinated water is its absorption by the hair and a resultant reaction forming Allworden sacs and bubbles that contain dissolved proteins of the upper cuticle layer (Bradbury & Leeder, 1970, p. 849; Fair & Gupta, 1987, p. 371). Thus, the sac formation renders hair weak, dry, dull, and with an unpleasant odor. Hair chemists have developed shampoos for the removal of chlorine from the hair, and the literature shows that the most successful system incorporates sodium thiosulfate in a general-purpose shampoo base in order to get rid of chlorine from the hair. This type of shampoo is very effective in combating the removal of chlorine from the hair. For wavy and curly/coily hair, the swimmers' shampoo base should be a detangling and moisturizing shampoo, which includes sodium thiosulfate as a chlorine-removing ingredient. To date, there is no swimmers' shampoo that prevents the penetration of chlorine into hair.

**Neutralizing/normalizing shampoos.** Neutralizing or normalizing shampoos are not commonly discussed in the literature. One reason for this is that general market companies do not market these types of shampoos. Neutralizing/normalizing shampoos bring the pH of the hair back to normal after chemical processes such as permanent coloring and bleaching since the pH of the hair during these processes is considerably high, 7-8. The general market trade may call a neutralizing shampoo an acidic shampoo, which does not quite eliminate alkaline residue from the hair and bring the hair pH back to its original state of 5-5.8. One reason for this gap in technology was the inability to measure the pH of the hair and scalp. However, over the last two decades, special pH meters have become available to measure the pH of the hair and scalp, enabling formulation chemists to develop neutralizing shampoos with precise control over normalizing the pH of hair after alkaline chemical treatments.

In the realm of textured hair, when wavy or curly/coily (Types 3 and 4) hair is relaxed by using relaxers containing active ingredients such as alkali metal hydroxides or guanidine hydroxide, the pH of the hair and scalp increases to ≈13 during relaxing. The pH of the hair and scalp drops down to ≈10 when these relaxers are rinsed from the hair. In order to neutralize the high alkaline pH of the hair and scalp, it is important that acidic shampoos with high neutralizing capacity are utilized to ensure that all of the alkaline remnants of relaxers are removed from the hair and scalp. Therefore, the pH of these shampoos should be in the range of 5-5.8.

pH is not the only issue that needs to be addressed after relaxer treatment; the damaged condition of the hair and scalp are also very important issues. Therefore, normalizing shampoos address all of the ill-effects of relaxers, whereas neutralizing shampoos merely balance the pH of the hair and scalp.

While formulating normalizing shampoos, chemists use a shampoo base consisting of a mixture of very mild detergents and co-detergents along with cationic conditioning agents such as polyquaternium-6, -7, or -10, mild organic acids, moisturizing ingredients, and strengthening materials such as fruit extracts or ceramides that will strengthen the hair and build back the stratum corneum of the scalp (Syed, 1997, p. 245). Other ingredients such as color indicators are added to signal that the hair and scalp are back to their original pH (Vermeulen, Banham, & Brooks, 2006, p. 483). Color indicators such as phenol red are not precise indicators that hair has reached its original pH. Antistatic agents are also included in the formulation in order to eliminate the buildup of a high electrostatic charge on the surface of chemically treated hair.

In order to formulate normalizing shampoos for straight or slightly wavy hair (Types 1 and 2) after permanent coloring or bleaching, the type and quantity of cationic polymers must be reduced significantly in order to avoid any polymeric buildup, which would contribute to a heavy feel, lack of bounce, and lack of free hair movement.

**Dry shampoos.** Dry shampoos do not contain detergents; they contain powders such as starch, silica, magnesium stearate, fragrance, and propellants. They are sprayed on dry hair to absorb sebum/oils from the hair and scalp. After spraying on the product, the hair is brushed, and the powder is removed by brushing. This product is ideal for quick shampooing without going through the process of wetting, lathering, rinsing, and drying the hair. Originally, this product was formulated with elderly and bedridden patients in mind. In recent decades, it has become popular for all consumers as an on-the-go shampoo when there is not enough time for wet shampooing, blow drying, and styling.

**Coloring shampoos.** The purpose of coloring shampoos is to enhance and increase the longevity of a particular shade that was applied previously using a semi-permanent color. Many shampoo formulas are developed that contain various colors in order to provide an array of color shades such as red, green, yellow, purple, blue, and more. Purple shampoos are also popular with bleach-blondes in order to remove brassiness from the bleached blonde hair. The base of these shampoos is the same as for moisturizing shampoos, which contain gentle detergents and moisturizing ingredients to compensate for the loss of moisture of color-treated hair and scalp, pH of the shampoo balanced to 5-5.8, hair strengthening ingredients such as ceramides, and other relevant additives.

## Conclusions

Human hygiene dictates that we cleanse our hair, scalp, and body on a regular basis. The cleansing of hair is not only a hygienic act, but also part of human beauty treatments. Humans express their beauty with cleansing, conditioning, and styling of the hair on a regular basis. However, the need of cleansing the hair and scalp is dependent on the type of hair and scalp one inherits. There are basic differences in the hair and scalp of humans based upon their ethnicity. When hair and scalp are oily or normal (Type 1), they need to be cleansed on a daily basis. On the other hand, when the hair is curly/coily (Types 3 and 4) and the scalp is dry, cleansing is practiced on a biweekly basis. The choice of shampoo is another crucial aspect for the health of the hair and scalp as well. Shampoos with higher concentrations of detergents may be needed to cleanse oily hair and scalp, while dry hair and scalp would need a shampoo containing gentler detergents such as amphoteric, non-ionic, and amino acid-derived detergents along with detangling, conditioning, and moisturizing additives, and pH balancing. This type of scalp would also be ideally set for a co-wash on a regular basis and further shampooing on a monthly basis. Dry-scalp consumers with dandruff will need a shampoo that contains one of the aforementioned anti-bacterial agents. Again, this shampoo should maintain the pH of hair and scalp in the range of 5-5.8 and not alter the natural moisture of the hair and scalp, and the stratum corneum of the scalp must stay unaltered.

# Exhibit A

## PRODUCT DEVELOPMENT REQUEST (PDR)

PDR No.: _____     PDR Date: _____

| | |
|---|---|
| Target introductory date: | |
| Product name: | |
| Product line: | |
| Product end user: | |

Category: <u>Radical</u>: Yes/No    <u>Incremental</u>: Yes/No    <u>Line Extension</u>: Yes/No

Initial screening of idea completed? Yes/No

Preliminary investigation completed? Yes/No

Detailed investigation of idea completed/business case developed? Yes/No

What are the perceived characteristics of the new product?

- *Relative advantage*: To what degree can this product be perceived as better than the product it supersedes?

- *Compatibility*: Is this product compatible with existing values, past experiences, and needs of potential adopters?

- *Observability*: Are the results of the product visible or demonstrable or communicable to others?

- *Complexity*: Is the product easy to use when compared to existing similar products?

- *Trial-ability*: Can this product be experimented with on a limited basis by the end user?

Sample PDR Form

## Exhibit A

| PRODUCT CHARACTERISTICS | REGULATORY REQUIREMENTS |
|---|---|
| Consistency:<br>Color:<br>Fragrance (describe):<br>pH:<br>Viscosity:<br>Description of packaging components: | The product is in compliance with:<br>· REACH, and Prop 65: Yes/No<br>· Food, Drug, and Cosmetic Act: Yes/No |
| **MAJOR COMPETITIVE BRANDS** | **COSTS** |
| Brand Name:<br>Size:<br>Salon List Price:<br>Salon Deal Price:<br>Consumer List Price:<br>Consumer Deal Price:<br>… | Ingredients cost per ounce or per fluid ounce:<br>Costs of container:<br>Costs of closure:<br>Costs of shipper:<br>Manufacturing costs:<br>Filling and packaging costs:<br>Any assembly costs:<br>Miscellaneous costs:<br>Total cost:<br><br>Is the cost viable for introduction of this product? Yes/No |

**PERSONNEL RESPOSIBLE FOR DEVELOPMENT**

| | |
|---|---|
| Idea Generator: | |
| Product Development Chemist: | |
| Vice President R&D: | |
| Marketing Product Manager: | |
| Vice President Marketing: | |
| President: | |

Sample PDR Form

# Exhibit A

**FOR LABORATORY USE**

| | |
|---|---|
| Formula No. after completion of the project: | |
| Estimated lab hours spent for the development of the product: | |
| Estimated hours spent on process development: | |
| New chemical purchases required: | |
| New lab and manufacturing equipment required: | |

*Approved by:*

_____    _____
Marketing Project Manager          Date

_____    _____
Development Chemist                Date

_____    _____
V.P. Mktg. & Sales                 Date

_____    _____
V.P. R&D                           Date

_____    _____
President                          Date

Sample PDR Form

## References

Agner, T., Damm, P., & Skouby, S. O. (1991). Menstrual cycle and skin reactivity. *Journal of the American Academy of Dermatology, 24*(4), 566–570.

Beauquey, B. (2005). Scalp and hair hygiene: Shampoos. In Bouillon & Wilkinson (Eds.), *The Science of Hair Care* (2nd ed.; pp. 83–127). Boca Raton, FL: Taylor & Francis.

Bradbury, J. H., & Leeder, J. D. (1970). Keratin fibers IV: Structure of cuticle. *Australian Journal of Biological Sciences, 23*, 843–854.

Berardesca, E., & Maibach, H. I. (1988). Racial differences in sodium lauryl sulfate-induced cutaneous irritation: Black and white. *Contact Dermatitis, 18*, 65–70.

Effendy, A., & Maibach, H. I. (1996). Detergent and skin irritation. *Clinics in Dermatology, 14*, 15–21.

Elsner. P., Wilhelm, D., & Maibach, H. I. (1991). Effect of low-concentration sodium lauryl sulfate on human vulvar and forearm skin: Age-related differences. *The Journal of Reproductive Medicine, 36*(1), 77–81.

Fair, N. B., & Gupta, B. S. (1987). The chlorine-hair interaction II: Effect of chlorination at varied pH levels on hair properties. *Journal of Society of Cosmetic Chemists, 38*, 371–384.

Faucher, J. A., & Goddard, E. D. (1978). Interaction of keratinous substrate with sodium lauryl sulfate: I. sorption. *Journal of the Society of Cosmetic Chemists, 29*(5), 323–337

Fortune Business Insights. (2019). https://www.globenewswire.com/news-release/2020/08/11/2076624/0/en/Shampoo-Market-Size-to-Reach-USD-37-92-Billion-by-2027-Increasing-Hair-Problems-among-Millennials-to-Fuel-Demand-states-Fortune-Business-Insights.html

Garcia, M. T., Campos, E., & Ribosa, I. (2007). Biodegradability and ecotoxicity of amine oxide-based surfactants. *Chemosphere, 69*, 1574–1578.

Gerstein, T. (1976). *Shampoo conditioner formulations.* United States Patent No. 3,990,991. Assignee: Revlon Inc. New York, NY. Washington, DC: United States Patent and Trademark Office.

Huang, H.-C., & Chang, T.-N. (2008). Ceramide 1 and ceramide 3 act synergistically on skin hydration and the transepidermal water loss of sodium lauryl sulfate-irritated skin. *International Journal of Dermatology, 47*, 812–819.

Imokawa, G., Akasaki, S., Minematsu, Y., & Kawai, M. (1989). Importance of intercellular lipids in water-retention properties of the stratum corneum: Induction and recovery study of surfactant dry skin. *Archives of Dermatological Research, 281*, 45–51.

Khalil, E., & Syed, A. N. (1980). *Low irritant conditioning shampoo composition.* United States Patent No. 4,205,063. Assignee: Johnson Products Co., Inc. Washington, DC: United States

Patent and Trademark Office.

Lewallen, R., Francis, S., Fisher, B., Richards, J., Li, J., Dawson, T., . . . & McMichael, A. (2015). Hair care practices and structural evaluation of scalp and hair shaft parameters in African-American and Caucasian women. *Journal of Cosmetic Dermatology, 14,* 216–223.

Markland, W. R. (1975). Shampoos. In deNavarre (Ed.), *The chemistry and manufacture of cosmetics* (2nd ed.; pp. 1283–1312). Orlando, FL: Continental Press.

Mizutani, T., Mori, R., Hirayama, M., Sagawa, Y., Shimizu, K., Okano, Y., & Masaki, H. (2016). Sodium lauryl sulfate stimulates the generation of reactive oxygen species through interactions with cell membranes. *Journal of Oleo Science, 65*(12), 993-1001

Schlossman, M. L. (2006). Bath and shower products. In Schlossman (Ed.), *The chemistry and manufacture of cosmetics* (3rd ed.; pp. 739–762). Carol Stream, IL: Allured

Schmid-Wendtner, M. H., & Korting, H. C. (2007). *pH and skin care.* Berlin, Germany: ABW Wissenschaftsverlag.

Sandhu, S. S., & Robbins, C. R. (1993). A simple and sensitive technique, based on protein loss measurements, to assess surface damage on human hair. *Journal of the Society of Cosmetic Chemists, 44*(2), 163–175.

Sandhu, S. S., Ramachandran, R., & Robbins, C. R. (1995). A simple and sensitive method using protein loss measurements to evaluate damage to human hair during combing. *Journal of the Society of Cosmetic Chemists, 46,* 39–52.

Smith, K. R., & Thiboutot, D. M. (2008). Sebaceous glands: Friend or foe? *Journal of Lipid Research, 49,* 271–281.

Smith, V. (2007). *Clean: A history of personal hygiene and purity.* Oxford, UK: Oxford University Press.

Sun, J. Z., Parr, W. A., & Erickson, M. C. E. (2003). Solubilization of sodium cocoyl isethionate. *Journal of Cosmetic Science, 54,* 559–568.

Syed, A. N. (1997). Ethnic hair care products. In D. Johnson (Ed.), *Hair and Hair Care* (pp. 235–259). New York, NY: Marcel Dekker.

Syed, A. N. (2008). *Bacteria growth on the African-descent scalp.* Avlon® Research Center, Unpublished Report No. 2008-01X, 1–6.

Syed, A. N., & Mathew, J. (2017). *The cleansing efficacy of sulfate-free shampoo and co-wash cleansing conditioners.* Avlon® Research Center. Unpublished Report No. 2017-01, 1–6.

Syed, A. N., Syed M. N., & Mathew, J. (2022). Texture Talk: Reinforcing Curly Hair Health. *Cosmetics & Toiletries Magazine, 137* (2), 46-56.

Syed, A. N., & Syed, M. N. (2017). *Textured hair: Its characteristics and comparison against nontextured hair.* SCC Symposium, October 12, 2017, New York, NY.

Syed, A. N., Hussain, M., & Hussain, A. (2008). *Acute skin response of commonly used detergents and their ranking using non-invasive bioengineering methods.* Avlon® Research Center. Unpublished Report No. 1- 8-2008, 1–107.

Syed, A. N., Kuhajda, A., Ayoub, H., Ahmad, K., & Frank, E. M. (1995, October). African-American hair: Its physical properties and differences relative to Caucasian hair. *Cosmetics & Toiletries Magazine, 110,* 39–48.

Syed, A. N., Ventura, T., & Syed, M. N. (2013). Hair ethnicity and ellipticity: A preliminary study. *Cosmetics & Toiletries Magazine, 128*(4), 250–259.

Vermeulen, S., Banham, A., & Brooks, G.J. (2006). Ethnic hair care. In Schlossman (Ed.), *The chemistry and manufacture of cosmetics* (3rd ed.; pp. 465–509). Carol Stream, IL: Allured.

Vie, K., Cours-Darne, S., Vienne, M. P., Boyer, F., Fabre, B., & Dupuy, P. (2002). Modulating effects of oatmeal extracts in the sodium lauryl sulfate skin irritancy model. *Skin Pharmacology and Applied Skin Physiology, 15,* 120–124.

Wong, M. (1997). Cleansing of hair. In Johnson (Ed.), *Hair and hair care* (pp. 33–64). New York, NY: Marcel Dekker.

# CHAPTER 6

# Conditioning & Damage Remedies

As the curvature of the hair changes from Type 1 to Type 4, the properties of the hair also change. Curvature can be defined as the degree to which a curve deviates from being a straight line. Type 1 hair has the least curvature, almost taking the shape of a straight line, whereas Type 4 hair has the most curvature. The higher the curvature of the hair, the greater is its waviness, curliness, or coiliness (Mettrie et al., 2007, p. 268). With this change in hair properties with increasing curvature, the conditioning needs of the hair also become different for each hair type.

Individuals with wavy, curly, and coily hair experience great difficulty in combing their hair. On average, it takes 15 to 16 minutes to detangle and comb wet curly/coily Type 4 hair, as compared to Type 1 hair, which can be combed in two to three minutes. This is one of the reasons that curly/coily hair consumers do not comb their hair on a daily basis. In fact, these consumers spend four to five hours grooming their hair on the day of shampooing due to the difficulties experienced with combing.

In **Table 3.1** of Chapter 3, the properties of Type 4 (curly/coily) hair were compared with those of Type 1 (straight) hair. It was concluded that Type 4 hair is very difficult to comb, has less moisture, less elasticity, less shine, a lower growth rate, higher ellipticity, higher porosity, more static charge, and more often a dry scalp beset with bacteria and fungi. Thus, to develop a high-quality conditioner for Type 3 and Type 4 hair, the formulating chemist must alleviate these hair and scalp issues. For example, conditioners for curlier hair types should ease combing difficulty, increase moisture, increase elasticity, decrease porosity, eliminate static charge, increase shine, rejuvenate the scalp for more hair growth, balance the pH of the hair and scalp, and eliminate harmful bacteria and fungi from the surface of the scalp. Before proceeding to resolve these issues though, the formulating chemist must understand the various causes of hair and scalp damage.

## Causes of Hair and Scalp Damage

Common sources of hair damage are shampooing, combing and brushing, weather-related phenomenon (e.g. UV radiation), thermal exposure, chlorine water in swimming pools, and chemical treatments. Each of these causes will be discussed below.

### Damage During Shampooing

Physical abrasion of wet hair is caused by rubbing movements of the fingers during sudsing of the shampoo. This rubbing action is responsible for cuticle damage or cuticle abrasion, and the cuticles are chipped away from the surface of the hair (Robbins, 2002, p. 193). Towel drying can also cause a small degree of damage to the hair due to rubbing movements. The detergents in shampoos can also remove structural lipids (p. 213). They can slowly but gradually dissolve a small portion of the non-keratinous cell membrane complex (CMC) and the endocuticles (Robbins, 1994, p. 154).

It was also observed that chemically treated hair, from alkaline treatments, can lose more cuticles during lathering with shampoos. Since the cuticles are somewhat loosely attached to the hair shaft of chemically treated hair in the alkaline state, they come apart or chip away easily from the hair shaft and float away in the sink during rinsing of the hair.

It is also recommended that wet hair, during and after shampooing, should be handled carefully with minimal manipulation. Combing after shampooing should be avoided unless appropriate conditioners are first applied for an appropriate length of time. Then, the hair may be combed, section by section, in thin partings. This technique leads to minimal damage.

### Combing and Brushing Damage

Combing and brushing are degradative processes for the hair, especially for Type 3 and Type 4 hair. During these processes, the hair is pulled repeatedly by applying considerable force, and the hair surface is constantly rubbed against by the teeth of the comb or bristles of the brush.

It has been reported that, during dry combing, the force needed to comb the hair is low at the root of the hair but increases tremendously as the comb moves toward the ends of the hair. Therefore, the ends of dry hair go through higher combing damage than the roots of dry hair for both short and long hair (Garcia, Epps, Yare, & Hunter, 1978, p. 172). These combing forces are even higher for African-descent, Type 3 and Type 4 hair (Syed et al., 1995, p. 46). Type 4 hair is even more affected during dry combing, as it is 32 times more difficult to comb than Type 1 hair (Syed & Syed, 2017, p. 21). Similarly, Type 4 wet hair requires 23 times more combing energy than Type 1 hair.

This excessive combing energy is significantly damaging to Type 4 hair because curly/coily hair extends over its elastic limits (Hookean region) when such a high combing energy is needed, and internal damage to the cortex takes place. For example, the hair loses up to 3-4% of its elasticity per 100 strokes of combing.

Combing and brushing after shampooing can damage the hair more than the lathering step of shampooing (Sandhu & Robbins, 1993, p. 39). Since the cuticles are somewhat loosely attached to the wet hair shaft, they come apart or chip away easily during combing. While the hair loses a great deal of its proteins, this loss can be significantly reduced by incorporating conditioning agents in shampoos and conditioners. Hair fibers treated with permanent waves, relaxers, and bleaches are even more susceptible to losing their cuticles during combing after shampooing (p. 51). However, the application of well-formulated conditioners can reduce the combing damage significantly, as the combing energy required to comb the hair is appreciably reduced through treatment with conditioners.

## Weather-Related Damage

The sun's heat and ultraviolet (UV) rays have a devastating effect on the hair. The heat generated by the sun dries out the hair, and UV rays alter and slightly bleach hair color. Heat and UV rays also change some of the cystine bonds into cysteic acid. This process results in weakening of the hair by decreasing its elasticity; the fibers become rigid or less flexible to bending during styling and grooming processes. Type 1 hair fibers, overexposed to UV light, are shown in **Figure 6.1**, where the cuticle layers of the hair fibers are completely fused or laminated together, making the hair rigid.

Solar-exposed hair loses its tensile strength and gloss and becomes somewhat dry due to the loss of its natural moisture. It also becomes raspy to the touch and difficult to comb in wet or dry states. The influence of weather becomes more obvious when individuals are wearing long hair and the hair at the ends become quite old. The ends of such hair show severe cuticular damage. They lose many of their cuticle layers because of wear and tear over the years. When combing, brushing, and solar damage combine, they make matters worse for the hair.

## Thermal Damage

Type 3 and Type 4 hair fibers have been heat treated for at least a century and a half. Early heat treatments dating back to the 1900s involved applying a pomade in conjunction with a hot metal comb that had been heated on the stove. This process was called pressing the hair (Syed et al., 1998, p. 47). Hair pressing was very common before the introduction of modern-day permanent hair relaxers, but even now, a small segment of the population still utilizes this process. Pressing aids in the form of creams are formulated from vegetable shortening and applied to the hair before the heat treatment. When the temperature of the hot comb reaches 230°C, the comb is passed through the hair three or four times to straighten the hair. In recent decades, the flat iron has taken the place of the pressing comb where the flatiron is passed through the hair for three to four passes to straighten the hair temporarily until the next cleansing with a shampoo. Regardless of whether a pressing comb or flat iron is used, this process is very damaging to hair, as the oils transfer the full brunt of the heat to the hair cortex, which becomes denatured, burns, and evaporates in smoke. The evidence of this mechanism is shown in **Figure 6.2** which shows a hair fiber whose cortex has been completely destroyed.

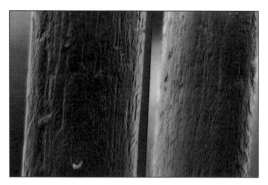

Figure 6.1. Scanning electron micrograph of Type 1 hair fibers exposed to UV light for 4 hours under 65% RH (x1550). Courtesy of Avlon® Research Center.

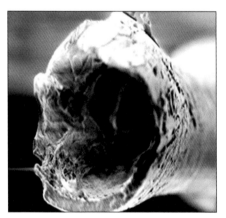

Figure 6.2. Scanning electron micrograph of a heat-treated hair fiber: (1) Vegetable shortening (natural vegetable oils) (2) 4 passes of a flat-iron at 230° C (x1550). Courtesy of Avlon® Research Center.

Thermal damage from blow-drying can occur as the heat from the blow-dryer drives out the inherent moisture of the hair. Furthermore, everyday use of blow-dryers and flat iron straighteners can cause serious structural damage to hair fibers. The inherent moisture of hair fibers converts to steam, which exerts pressure on the walls of the cuticle layers from inside the cortex. Consequently, the cuticle layers burst open causing radial cracks in the fiber, as depicted in **Figure 6.3**. The radial cracks are further insulted during combing and brushing by the teeth of the comb or the bristles of the brush, making them even larger in size. Eventually, the hair fiber will break into pieces on repeated grooming practices. Normally, fiber elasticity decreases by 18% if no thermal protectants are used during blow-drying and flat ironing. Radial cracks and decreased elasticity can be minimized significantly, and elasticity loss may decrease to only 6% if proper thermal protectants, based on volatile silicones, are used prior to thermal treatment.

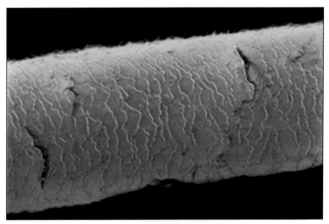

Figure 6.3. Scanning electron mircrograph (x800) of a hair fiber treated with 7 passes of a flat-iron set at 204° C. Radial cracks are visible along the hair shaft. Courtesy of Avlon® Research Center.

## Chlorinated-Water Damage of Swimmers' Hair

Allworden (as cited in Fair & Gupta, 1987) studied the damaging effect of large concentrations of chlorine in water on wool fibers. Much later, the effect of chlorinated water was investigated on human hair at the parts-per-million level to simulate the effect of chlorine in swimming pools on hair (p. 371). The researchers measured the effect of chlorinated water in terms of increase in hair friction properties and fiber strength. Hair friction did increase significantly even at the parts per million level of chlorine at pH 2 and 7, whereas the increase in hair friction was lowest at pH 10. The friction of hair also increased with more treatments of hair with chlorinated water. Fiber strength also decreased significantly as the number of treatment cycles increased, both at pH 2 and 7, but the fiber strength did not decrease at pH 10. The ill effects of chlorinated water on hair in terms of increased friction and decreased fiber strength are negligible at pH 10 (p. 383). When the hair fibers are treated with chemicals such as bleaches, dyes, and permanent waves, the impact of chlorinated water on chemically treated hair increases the interfiber friction, affects the cuticular morphology, and decreases the hair fiber weight (Fair & Gupta, 1988, p. 104).

## Damage From Chemical Treatments

Many consumers treat their hair with reactive chemicals such as relaxers, permanent colors, hair lighteners, permanent waves, and smoothing treatments containing formaldehyde or glyoxylic acid. Along with chemically damaging the hair, these chemical treatments change the chemical and physical structure of the hair fibers permanently. Damage appears in the form of losing a significant number of cuticles, fiber elasticity, natural surface oil (18-MEA), cuticular CMC, some cortex proteins, and moisture of the hair and scalp, as well as through increased inflammation and irritation of the scalp and lost integrity of the stratum corneum of the scalp. Porosity of the chemically treated fibers increases, and the hair becomes more sensitive to humidity and less manageable in hot humid climates. Under low humidity conditions, hair becomes dry and brittle.

One way to eliminate chemical damage is to avoid chemical treatments altogether. Since 2005, there has been a strong movement in the marketplace, where consumers with Type 3 and Type 4 hair have stopped using chemical treatments to avoid chemical damage. These consumers are now styling their hair in its natural state. The trade-off here is that they spend significantly more time maintaining and styling their curly/coily hair every week, which can be tiring and sometimes frustrating. However, they still visit hair salons for haircuts, deep conditioning, proper hair care instructions for naturally styling hair, and other services.

Some consumers with naturally wavy, curly, or coily hair may still opt for certain chemical treatments such as permanent hair coloring and permanent hair lightening to enhance the look of their hair and, in the case of older consumers, to conceal gray hair. Of course, chemical damage still takes place with these treatments, but the damage can be graded. After permanent color treatment, hair loses about 6% elasticity (Syed & Ayoub, 2002, p. 60). Particularly, bright red shades of permanent colors can decrease hair elasticity up to 20%. The hair and scalp lose moisture, and other associated damage may result such as cuticle reduction, loss of some 18-MEA, and increase in porosity of 3-4% for color-treated hair (p. 60). In case of hair lightening, the loss of fiber elasticity is close to 25% (p. 60), along with other losses in the moisture of the hair and scalp, number of cuticle layers, and amount of 18-MEA. The porosity of the hair increases most upon hair lightening (p. 60). Additionally, the hair loses some of its curl pattern and becomes very unruly and unmanageable during lightening. Lightened hair of Types 3 & 4 is extremely difficult to comb and breaks easily upon combing and brushing. In fact, hair lightening is the most damaging chemical treatment, even more so than hair relaxer treatment.

## Remedies for Hair Damage

To reduce or eliminate hair and scalp damage, conditioning agents are utilized in the form of hair and scalp conditioners. These conditioners can be categorized into the chemical classes of quaternary ammonium compounds, cationic polymers, and silicones. Each of these classes will be discussed below before positioning them to alleviate various types of damage for different types of hair and scalp.

### Class 1.0. Quaternary Compounds

Quaternary ammonium compounds (quats) are a class of conditioning agents that bear a positive charge and can attach to the negative sites of the hair fiber. Hair fibers normally have equal degrees of positive and negative charges, but the negative charge increases as hair fiber damage increases. The more damaged the hair fiber, the greater the presence of negative charges. Therefore, positively charged quaternary compounds are attracted to damaged negative sites on the hair and attach themselves to the damaged sites, thereby helping to repair and condition the hair. Hair chemists have many quaternary ammonium compounds at their disposal. The specific quat that is used will depend on hair type (i.e. Types 1-4) and the need of the hair.

### Class 1.1. Quaternary Ammonium Compounds with Monoalkyl Groups from $C_{16}$-$C_{22}$

Simple quaternary ammonium compounds are formed when tertiary amines or ethoxylated amines are alkylated with metal halides or dimethyl sulfate. The structure of a monoalkyl quaternium compound is presented in **Figure 6.4**. The conditioning profile of a quaternium compound depends on the length of the carbon chain and the number of alkyl groups (Jurczyk et al., 1991, p. 65). The lower the carbon chain length, the less conditioning or ease of combing of hair will result. Similarly, the longer the carbon chain length of the alkyl group, the more hydrophobic effect on the hair results; hence, more ease of combing.

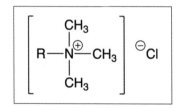

Figure 6.4. Structure of monoalkyl trimethyl ammonium chloride, where -R represents an alkyl group anywhere from 12 to 22 carbons in length.

The alkyl groups can also be ethoxylated, which may help rinse off the quaternary compounds from the hair. Quaternary ammonium compounds consisting of alkyl chains of 8-10 carbons in length are known to be germicidal and fungicidal.

Monoalkyl quaternium compounds are well-suited for Type 1 and Type 2 hair, but Types 3 and 4 hair will need the addition of other quaternary compounds with long carbon chain dialkyl groups in order to attain the most effective conditioning. It is also customary to include more than one conditioning agent to obtain the desired conditioning properties in a hair conditioner depending upon the condition of the hair such as color-treated, bleached, dry, or oily hair.

Some examples of these compounds are cetyl trimonium chloride, stearyl trimonium chloride, and behentrimonium chloride, where the R group can range from C16-C22. Cetyl trimonium chloride is also called cetrimonium chloride; it foams well and can be used as a surface-active agent in addition to acting as a conditioner. It is more suited for fine-textured, Type 1 hair.

### Class 1.2. Quaternary Ammonium Compounds with Dialkyl Groups from $C_{16}$-$C_{22}$

Quaternary ammonium compounds that contain two alkyl groups (**Figure 6.5**) impart better conditioning properties to Type 3 and Type 4 hair. These compounds are dispersible in water.

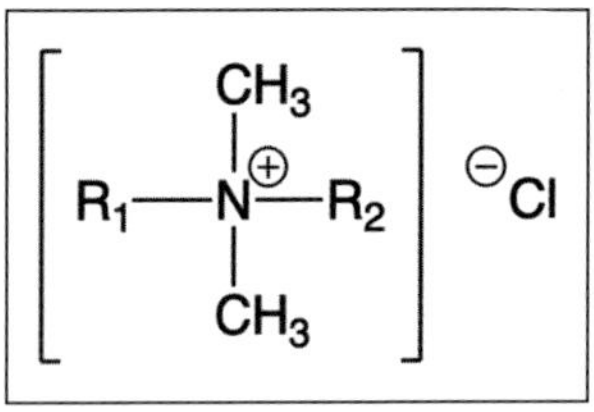

$$\left[ R_1 - \overset{\overset{CH_3}{|}}{\underset{\underset{CH_3}{|}}{N^{\oplus}}} - R_2 \right] \ ^{\ominus}Cl$$

**Figure 6.5.** Structure of dialkyl dimethyl ammonium chloride. -$R_1$ and -$R_2$ represent alkyl groups 16 to 22 carbons in length.

The conditioning properties of dialkyl quaternary ammonium compounds are more suitable for wavy, curly/coily hair because these Class 1.2 compounds have longer alkyl chain lengths and a higher number of alkyl groups. The kinetics of adsorption also varies depending on the alkyl chain length and number of alkyl groups. Quaternary ammonium compounds form micelles and adsorb onto the surface of hair forming a thin, permeable layer. A micelle is a molecular aggregate of 50 to 100 molecules that form colloidal particles. Micelle formation is dependent upon the alkyl chain length and concentration of the quaternary ammonium compound.

The longer the alkyl carbon chain of a quaternary compound, the milder the compound will be to the skin and the less irritating to the eyes. Therefore, $C_{20-22}$ alkyl (behenyl) groups in quaternary compounds are very gentle to the skin and do not cause eye irritation. Behenyl and longer chain alkyl groups are used on Type 3 and Type 4 hair, damaged hair, and for deep conditioning. However, these longer chain groups can make Type 1 (Caucasian) hair feel heavy. Such conditioners should be used on a weekly or biweekly basis, rather than daily (Hoshowski, 1997, p. 73). Similarly, ditallow ammonium compounds are effective conditioners for wavy and curly/coily Types 3 and 4 hair (Syed, 1997, p. 254). Examples of compounds in this class are dicetyldimonium chloride, distearyldimonium chloride, dimethyl di-(hydrogenated tallow) ammonium chloride (quaternium-18), and dibehenyl ammonium chloride.

Class 1.3. Ester Quats

Initially, ester quat technology was developed for fabric softeners in the year 2000. These compounds are now being positioned as hair conditioners. Ester quats contain ester groups instead of alkyl fatty groups, although the R in the -RCO group still represents a fatty group from tallow, palmitic, coco acids, or any other long carbon chain fatty acid. Ester quats are available as mono- and diester forms for conditioning the hair. One example of a monoester quat is quaternium-87; its structure shown in **Figure 6.6**.

As compared to monoester quats, diester quats are particularly suited for Types 3 and 4 hair. Several examples of diester quats will be given. The first example is quaternium-82 (see **Figure 6.7** for structure). In this diester quat, two -RCO groups are present; they are derived from the fatty acid, oleic acid. These diester quaternium compounds confer great

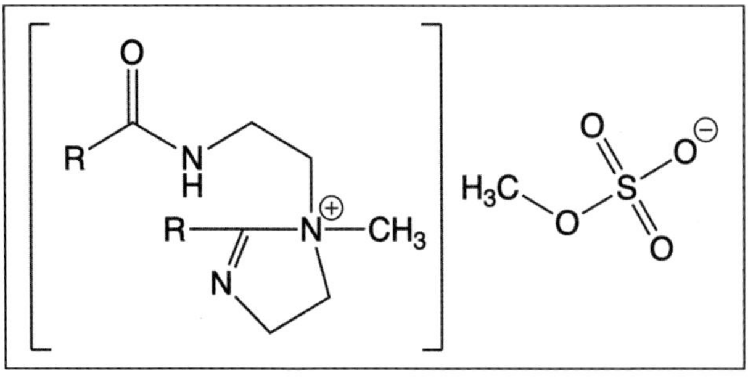

Figure 6.6. Structure of quaternium-87, which is a monoester quat. The -RCO and -R groups are derived from palm oil.

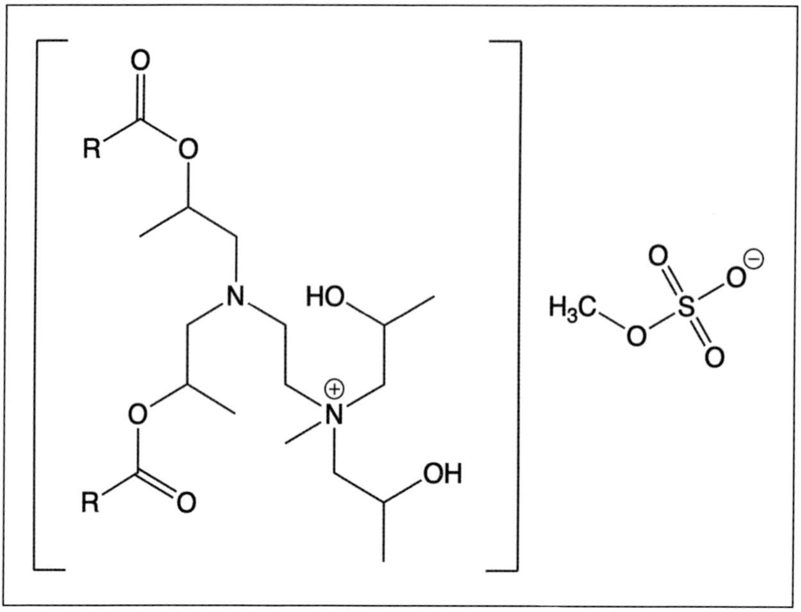

**Figure 6.7.** Structure of quaternium-82, which is a diester quat. The -RCO and -R groups are derived from oleic acid.

ease of combing to wavy, curly/coily Type 3 and Type 4 hair during wet and dry combing. These quats may make fine, limp, Type 1 hair less manageable and feel oily and greasy.

The second example of a diester quat is quaternium-53 whose structure is shown in **Figure 6.8**. The two -RCO groups represent tallow

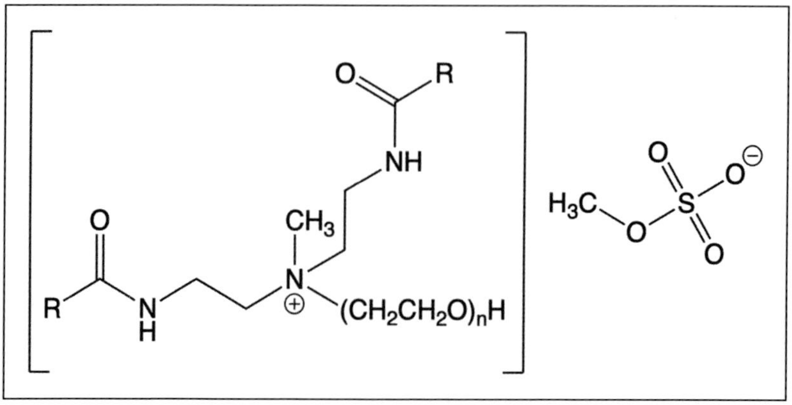

**Figure 6.8.** Structure of quaternium-53, consisting of two -RCO groups that represent tallow acid radicals.

acid esters. Quaternium-53 also makes wavy, curly/coily Type 3 and Type 4 hair very easy to comb as compared to Class 1.1 and 1.2 quaternary ammonium compounds. **Figure 6.9** depicts the structure of a dialkyl ester quat derived from triethanolamine. The ester group, -RCO, may be derived from palm oil in one example or tallow in another example.

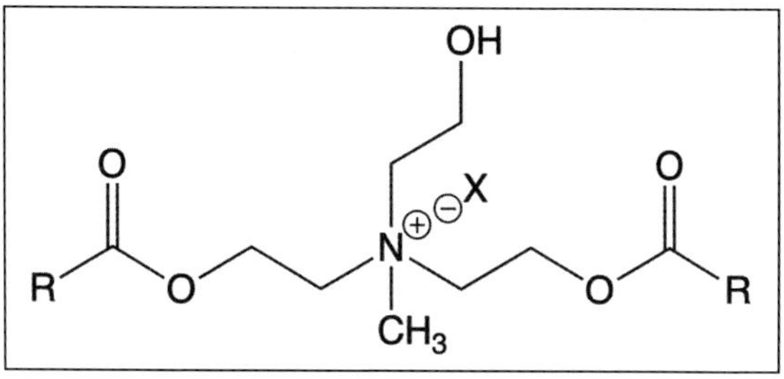

Figure 6.9. Structure of a diester quat derived from triethanolamine where X- is the counter anion. The -RCO groups may be derived from tallow or palm oil.

## Class 2.0. Silicone-Based Polymers

Numerous polymers of the silicone family act as conditioning agents. They may or may not possess a positive charge, but they condition the hair in terms of ease of combing, elimination of static electricity, increasing shine, improving fiber elasticity, and other improvements. Examples of common silicones are discussed in the following sections.

### Class 2.1. Dimethicones

Dimethicones are a type of uncharged, silicone-based polymer that possess a repeat unit consisting of a -SiO moiety connected to three methyl groups, [-(CH3)-Si-O]. The general structure of a dimethicone polymer is shown in **Figure 6.10**. The degree of polymerization tells us how many re-

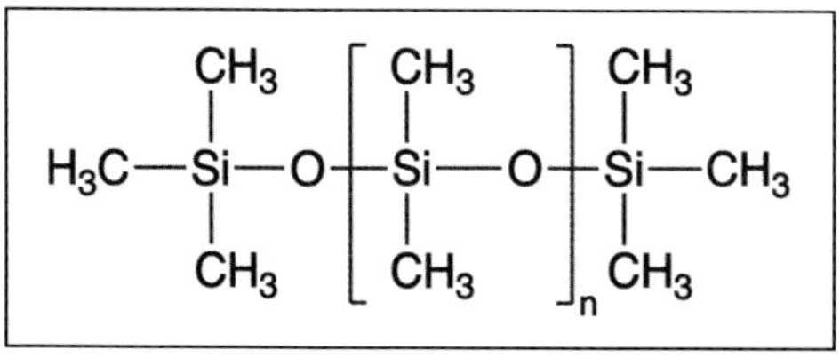

Figure 6.10. Structure of dimethicone polymer. The number of n units varies to form various types of dimethicones with differing properties.

peat units [-(CH3)-Si-O] are connected to form the dimethicone chain. The higher the degree of polymerization, the larger the size of the dimethicone polymer, and the higher its viscosity. Dimethicones are non-polar, hydrophobic, and have a low surface energy, which makes them excellent water repellents and good lubricants for the surface of the hair. In turn, these polymers impart ease of wet and dry combing and help smoothen the cuticles. Dimethicones are water-insoluble and are added to conditioning formulations in order to increase the ease of combing for hard-to-comb hair. These compounds are somewhat difficult to remove from the hair through shampooing; they may last on the hair surface through as many as four or five shampooing treatments.

Dimethicones have become unpopular among consumers with Type 3 and Type 4 hair because of the difficulty of rinsing these silicones out from the hair. Thus, as you continuously use silicones on your hair, buildup can accumulate easily, leading to unfavorable hair conditions. For these reasons, naturalistas, a group of consumers who prefer to maintain natural hair and to use natural products, refrain from using products that contain dimethicones or any type of silicone.

Class 2.2. Amino-Functional Silicone Polymers

When the methyl groups ($-CH_3$) of dimethicone are replaced with amino groups ($-NH_2$), aminofunctional silicones are formed. In acidic environments, such as those of a conditioner, they bear a positive charge at the -N site and thus have a great affinity for the negative (damaged) sites on the hair fiber. Aminofunctional silicones are called amodimethicones. The structure of these compounds is shown in **Figure 6.11**. Like dimethicones, amodimethicones have become unpopular among consumers with Type 3 and Type 4 hair, by virtue of being silicones. Amodimethicones avoid the buildup issues of other silicones though because they bear a positive charge. Thus, amodimethicone layers repel each other and do not form thick silicone layers, as dimethicones do for example.

## Class 3.0. Homo- and Copolymers

The use of synthetic cationic polymers is very popular in hair care products such as shampoos, conditioners, and styling products. Cationic

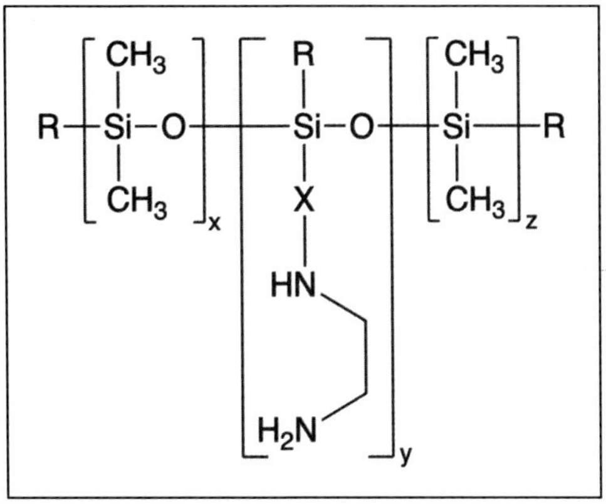

**Figure 6.11.** Structure of an amodimethicone polymer, where R is OH or $CH_3$, and X represents either a propyl, isopropyl, or isobutyl group.

polymers are of two types: homopolymers and copolymers.

**Polyquaternium-10** is one of the most widely used cationic polymers in shampoos and conditioners as it adsorbs readily onto proteinaceous surfaces, such as hair and skin. Polyquaternium-10 is a copolymer quaternary ammonium salt of hydroxyethyl cellulose reacted with a trimethyl ammonium substituted epoxide. Its structure is shown in **Figure 6.12**. It is commonly added to detangling 2-in-1 shampoos, and to conditioners for hard-to-comb Types 3 and 4 hair, to make wet and dry combing easier

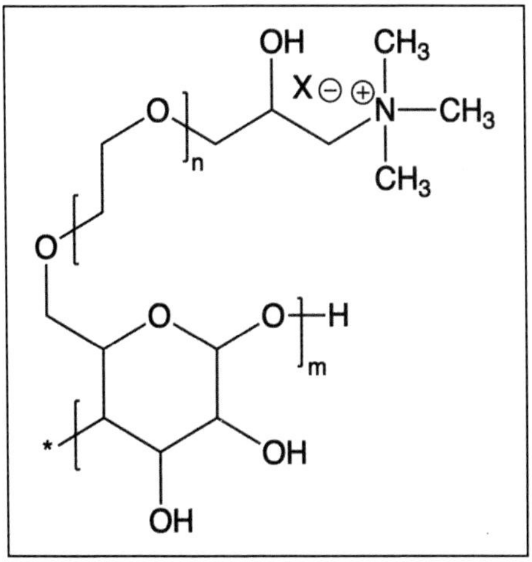

**Figure 6.12.** Structure of polyquaternium-10. The subscripts m and n denote the degree of polymerization of hydroxyethyl cellusose and the epoxide respectively. X represents the counter anion, usually $Cl^-$.

and reduce combing damage. This polymer is also used in wet-setting hair preparations, where wet hair is rolled on rollers with a setting lotion and then dried.

**Polyquaternium-6** is a homopolymer of diallydimethyl ammonium chloride (DADMAC). The structure of polyquaternium-6 is shown in **Figure 6.13**. To synthesize polyquaternium-6, first allylchloride and dimethylamine are reacted to form DADMAC. Next, DADMAC is polymerized in aqueous solution utilizing an organic peroxide catalyst. This polymer has a high cationic charge and is very effective in conditioning the hair. Thus it is incorporated in many types of hair care products, including 2-in-1 shampoos, hair relaxers, pre-chemical conditioners, and post-chemical conditioners.

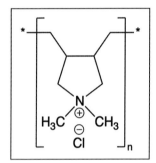

Figure 6.13. Structure of polyquaternium-6. The subscript n denotes the degree of polymerization.

**Polyquaternium-7** is also widely used in the hair care industry, specifically in shampoos and conditioners. It is a copolymer of dimethyl

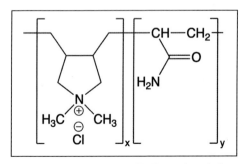

Figure 6.14. Structure of polyquaternium-7. The subscripts x and y denote the degree of polymerization of each monomer.,

diallyl ammonium chloride and acrylamide (see **Figure 6.14** for structure).

**Polyquaternium-11** is used in setting wet hair to a desired shape with a clear, glossy film on the hair. It is a copolymer of vinylpyrrolidone and dimethylamine ethylmethacrylate, partially quaternized with diethyl sulfate. The structure of Polyquaternium-11 is shown in **Figure 6.15**.

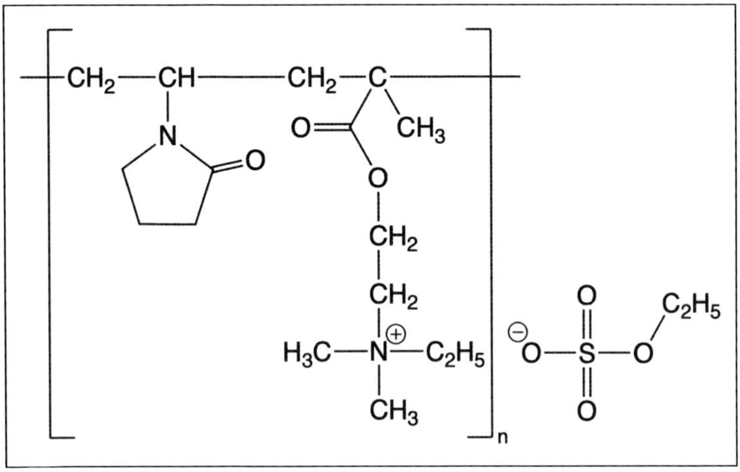

Figure 6.15. Structure of polyquaternium-11. The subscript n denotes the degree of polymerization.

## State of Hair & Scalp Before Conditioner Treatment

After exposure to various damage factors and before treatment with a conditioner, the state of the hair and scalp may be in any of the following conditions:

- Hair fibers are hard to comb after cleansing with shampoo.
- Hair fibers may have lost some cuticles, cuticular CMC, and cuticular lipids from shampooing damage.
- Cuticles are worn out due to combing and brushing damage.
- Cuticles are swollen and open from exposure to harsh deter-

gents of shampoos and chemical damage.

- Hair fibers lost elasticity from chemical treatments and combing and brushing of hard-to-comb hair.
- Porosity of hair fibers increased due to combing, brushing, and chemical treatments.
- Hair fibers are damaged and become dry with lack of moisture and are raspy in feel from chemical treatments.
- Hair is shedding and thinning either due to scalp conditions or excessive chemical damage.
- The scalp is turning over cells that generate bacteria and fungi on the scalp.
- The pH of the hair and scalp are elevated and need to be regulated to 5-5.8.
- Stratum corneum of the scalp has increased TEWL.
- Hair has solar damage due to exposure to ultraviolet rays.
- Cuticles are damaged by chlorinated water in swimming pools.
- Buildup of calcium and magnesium ions from hard water on hair fiber surface.
- Hair and scalp have buildup from various pollutants.

## Factors Influencing Penetration of Conditioners

In order to mitigate the aforementioned damage, various types of conditioners must be formulated. Before discussing how to the alleviate damage to the hair and scalp by using conditioners, it is important to know how to effectively penetrate conditioners into the hair and scalp. Three main factors influence the penetration of conditioners:

1. Length of treatment time
2. Heat
3. pH of hair

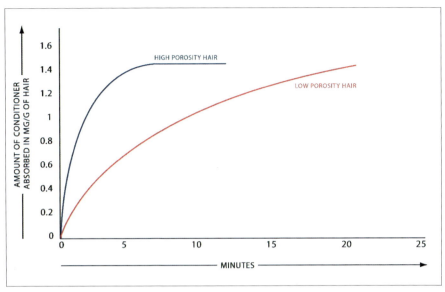

Figure 6.16. The amount of conditioner absorbed into the hair (mg/g of hair) versus time (minutes). Data for high porosity hair and low porosity hair.

Each of these factors will be discussed below.

## Length of treatment time

The treatment time of a conditioner should be the time required for the conditioner to penetrate the hair and scalp. The relationship between the amount of conditioner absorbed into the hair for both high and low porosity hair over time is shown in **Figure 6.16**. For a few minutes initially, there is a linear relationship between application time and the amount of conditioner absorbed by the hair, which reaches a maximum and then, plateaus after a certain length of time, called the *optimum application time*. The amount of absorbed conditioner also depends on the porosity of the hair. If the hair is porous, it takes less time for the absorption of the conditioner (Lotzsch, Reng, Gantz, & Quack, 1981, p. 645). On the other hand, if hair porosity is low, the absorption time increases significantly. Normally, a good conditioner can penetrate the hair in 15 to 20 minutes. In some cases, if the hair has low porosity, it may take 30 minutes for a conditioner to penetrate the cortex.

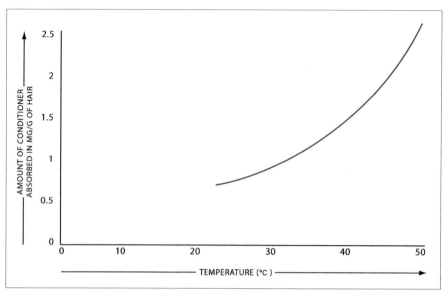

Figure 6.17. The amount of conditioner absorbed into the hair (mg/g of hair) versus temperature (°C).

## Heat

If a consumer is pressed for time, a combination of heat and time can help cut down on the total time taken to condition the hair. Also, if the conditioning molecule, meaning, the quaternary compound, is large in its molecular size, it would take longer for the conditioner to penetrate the hair. Therefore, it is advisable to use both time and heat, if available, to deep-condition the hair (see **Figure 6.17**). At home, the consumer can leave the conditioner on her hair for up to an hour without a heat source for deeper conditioner penetration. If a heat source (e.g. hooded dryer, thermal heat cap, hot towel wrap, steamer, etc.) is used, it may take only 20 to 25 minutes for low porosity hair to absorb most of the conditioner. The hair should be allowed to cool down for 5 minutes before rinsing the conditioner from the hair. It is important to note that when applying heat to the hair, it should be done carefully to avoid causing damage to the hair or scalp. The heat source should be applied for a limited amount of time and at a safe temperature to prevent overheating or burning the hair or scalp.

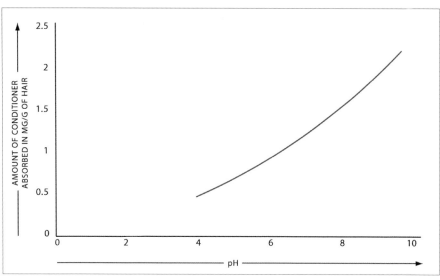

**Figure 6.18.** The amount of conditioner absorbed into the hair (mg/g of hair) as a function of hair pH.

## pH of hair

The pH of the hair is elevated during chemical treatments such as permanent hair coloring, permanent hair lightening (bleaches), permanent waves, and permanent hair relaxers. During chemical treatments, the pH of the hair increases in relation to the pH of the specific product being applied. For example, the pH of hair increases to ~10 when applying a hair lightener or a permanent color; similarly, the pH of hair increases to ~13 during relaxing with sodium hydroxide or guanidine hydroxide relaxers. The cuticles of the hair are wide open during these alkaline treatments. Although hair is in its most vulnerable state under these conditions, the opportunity for cationic polymers to penetrate deep into the cortex layer of the hair is at its greatest. When cuticles are closed, it is difficult for conditioners to penetrate deep into the cortex. If they do, an extended amount of time is required. Therefore, if a special cationic polymer is applied to the hair before the chemical treatment, the cationic molecule penetrates deeper into the hair. This conditioning is more permanent and can stay in the hair for up to four shampoo treatments. Conditioning at elevated pH cannot be accomplished with just any conditioner as most of the conditioning ingredients are rendered ineffective at high alkaline pH. Therefore, a special class of cationic polymers such as polyquaternium-6 and cationic polyamines that are stable at high alkaline pH are used for this purpose. They can condition the hair while a chemical treatment is on the hair (Hsuing & Mueller, 1979, Col. 5; Syed, 1986, col. 12; Syed & Ahmad, 1997, col. 14).

Even when the chemicals are first rinsed from the hair, the pH declines only partially (down to ~9.5-10 with relaxers, ~8 with hair lighteners). The hair is still alkaline, and the cuticles remain partially open. This represents the second-best opportunity to condition the hair before completely closing the cuticles with normalizing/acidic shampoos.

Shown in **Figure 6.18**, the relationship of pH and the penetration of a conditioner has been reported where the amount of conditioner penetrating the hair increases as the pH of the hair increases (Lotzch et al., 1981, p. 646).

## Types of Conditioners

Before conditioning the hair, the specific type of hair damage must be diagnosed. Once identified, a damage remedy in terms of conditioning can be prescribed. In order to eliminate or alleviate various types of damage to hair, different types of conditioners are applied to hair under specific conditions. The varying forms of conditioners are as follows:

- Pre-chemical conditioners
- Post-chemical conditioners
- Leave-in conditioner for natural Type 3 and Type 4 hair
- Leave-in conditioner for relaxed hair
- Moisturizing conditioners
- Anti-dandruff conditioner
- Deep-penetrating conditioners
- Damage-repair conditioners based on cross-linking technology
- Reconstructive conditioners
- Anti-thinning and anti-shedding hair conditioners

- Conditioners for color-treated hair
- Coloring conditioners
- Blow-drying lotion/conditioners
- Laminate for thermal damage reduction
- Anti-frizz conditioners

**Pre-Chemical Conditioners**

Pre-chemical conditioners are relatively new to the marketplace. The first conditioner in this category was formulated in 1985 to condition hair before and during relaxer treatment. A mixture of conditioning agents such as cationic polyamines (Syed, 1986, col. 14) and positively charged macromolecules (Syed & Ahmad, 1997, col. 12) were applied to the hair before chemical treatment and left on the hair during the chemical application. As the hair swelled during chemical treatment at pH 10 or 13, these large molecules were able to penetrate the hair cortex. These molecules

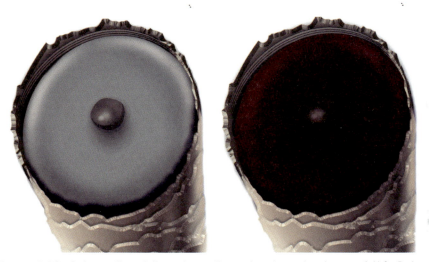

Figure 6.19. Schematic of the absorption of polyquaterniums of U.S. Patent 5,639,449. The left side depicts the before state of the hair. After treatment with pre-chemical conditioner and relaxer, the hair was rinsed and treated with the Rubin dye test to detect the presence of cationic polymers. The schematic on the right side shows that the cortex contained cationic polyquaterniums, represented by the red color in the cortex.

were stable at high pH. While rinsing off the chemical, the hair started to deswell, and many of these large, bulky conditioning molecules stayed inside the cortex of the hair, significantly (see **Figure 6.19**).

This procedure represents a more permanent conditioning and lasts for up to four shampoo treatments. These conditioning molecules are able to facilitate ease of combing in both the wet and dry states, and increase the tensile strength of the hair fiber.

## Post-Chemical Conditioners

Post-chemical conditioners were first introduced in the mid-1980s, where the concoction contained a cationic polymer such as polyquaternium-10, proteins, detergents, and a high concentration of hydrochloric acid (Syed & Gross, 1986, column 4). This formulation had a pH of 2.5 and was applied to the hair for five minutes after rinsing out the relaxer. The pH of the hair was ~10 when the relaxer/hair straightener was rinsed from the hair and the cuticles were still partially open. It is, therefore, the second most opportune time for the cationic polymers and other active agents to penetrate the cortex. The absorption of cationic polymers increased, and the hair became much easier to detangle and comb. The drawback of such post-chemical solutions was the inclusion of detergents and exclusion of lipids, which made the hair and scalp dry with lack of moisture. The next generation of post-chemical conditioners were developed by this author; they were cream based and contained not only cationic polymers but also a higher dose of gentle organic acids as alkali neutralizers, conditioning agents, proteins, fruit extracts, and ceramides. These cream-based post-chemical conditioners brought the pH of the hair and scalp back into the neutral pH range, minimized combing damage, and increased fiber elasticity. These cream-based post-chemical conditioners have become the benchmark for the industry; they are also used after rinsing hair colors or hair bleaches from the hair.

## Leave-In Conditioners

There are two versions of leave-in conditioners: One version is suited for natural Type 3 and Type 4 hair, while the second version is more suitable for chemically relaxed Type 3 and Type 4 hair.

**Leave-In Conditioners for Natural Type 3 and Type 4 hair.** After cleansing Type 3 and Type 4 hair with either a shampoo or co-wash, the hair is treated with a leave-in conditioner. This conditioner contains humectants such as glycerin, quaternary compounds such as behentrimonium chloride or methosulfate and others, moisturizing agents, emulsifiers, organic acids for pH adjustment, and safe preservatives. Usually, this emulsion is of medium viscosity, easy to apply to naturally curly hair, and easily spreadable on the hair. After the application of the leave-in conditioner, the hair is combed and ready for the application of styling-aids. It is important that the hair is sprayed with water or Coconut Oil or Jamaican Black Castor Oil Water to keep it wet during styling to avoid any flaking of the styling products on the hair in the dry state. It takes approximately 45 minutes to 1 hour to style the hair either by the strand twist method or the wash & go method. In each case, consumers use their fingers to either twist the hair or twirl it into a coil formation. If the hair starts to dry out during styling, it is advisable to spray it with Coconut Oil Water or Jamaican Black Castor Oil Water.

**Leave-In Conditioners for Chemically Modified Hair.** These conditioners are applied to the hair after relaxing and before blow-drying and flat ironing. A small amount of quaternium compounds such as quaternium-18 or behentrimonium methosulfate or chloride or any other quaternium compounds are used in the emulsion. Similarly, a small quantity of oil, ultraviolet absorbers, volatile silicones such as thermal protectants, ceramides, and other strengthening ingredients, such as hydrolyzed keratin or hydrolyzed wheat proteins, are also included in this emulsion. The concentration of oils must be optimized to avoid making the hair oily. Such conditioners make combing very easy. They strengthen the hair, help protect it from heat appliances, and help replenish lost proteins and lipids from the cuticle layers of the hair fibers.

## Moisturizing Conditioners

This category of conditioners is marketed to consumers with dry hair. These conditioners contain quaternium compounds with long chain alkyl groups such as behenyl or tallow, moisturizing ingredients such as glycerin, glycereth-26, and fruit extracts such as beet root extract, which are hygroscopic in nature. The pH of the formulation is adjusted to 5-5.8 to provide a healthy hair and scalp environment. Other ingredients such as ceramides are also added to maintain the stratum corneum of the scalp with respect to transepidermal water loss.

## Anti-Dandruff Conditioners

Anti-dandruff conditioners are formulated to remove dandruff flakes from the scalp and condition the hair and scalp. The continuous use of an anti-dandruff shampoo followed by an anti-dandruff conditioner helps to manage scalp dandruff. If use is discontinued, the dandruff will reappear within six weeks. FDA/REACH approved active anti-dandruff ingredients are zinc pyrithione, selenium sulfide, ketoconazole, sulfur, salicylic acid, among others. Normally, zinc pyrithione is added to the conditioner base at a 0.50-1.0% active level, along with moisturizing ingredients to moisturize dry hair and scalp. The pH of the conditioner is adjusted to 5-5.8 with organic acids.

## Deep-Penetrating Conditioners

These conditioners are formulated primarily to condition severely damaged hair that has been treated with multiple chemicals and is overprocessed. In deep conditioners, many different types of ingredients are added at optimum levels such as quaternium compounds, moisturizers, fiber strengtheners, anti-static agents, porosity reducers, and other damage-mitigating ingredients to accomplish the various elements of hair conditioning. For example, upon treating the hair with these conditioners for 15 to 20 minutes, the hair develops the following characteristics:

- Easy to comb in both the wet and dry state
- Increased moisture
- Cuticles show reduced swelling and are repaired in terms of their lost proteins and lipids from combing damage

- Increased elasticity
- Hair does not develop static electricity upon repeated combing
- Hair loss during combing is minimized
- Reduced porosity
- Enhanced shine
- More body
- The pH of the hair is balanced to 5-5.8
- The hair fibers feel perceptibly stronger
- Any hard-water buildup of calcium and magnesium is removed

**Damage-Repair Conditioners Based on Cross-Linking**

Recent developments in conditioning technologies has allowed for the cross-linking of broken bonds of the hair, such as cysteine -SH, with the use of glycidoxy silicones (Syed & Olenick, 2019). Other advancements are liquid crystalline systems and submicron emulsions, which reduce the particle size of an emulsion to the nanometer (nm) scale. A nanometer is one billionth of a meter. Normally, emulsion particles are 10 to 20 microns in size (a micron is one millionth of a meter). In a submicron emulsion, the particles are reduced to ~200 to 800 nm in size. These smaller particles penetrate deeper into the hair, thereby producing more permanent conditioning of the hair. The rest of the ingredients are similar to deep-penetrating conditioners.

## Reconstructive Conditioners

Reconstructive conditioners are intended to rebuild severely damaged hair. The term "reconstructive" may be a misnomer though because permanently damaged hair cannot be brought back to its original state. Damaged hair can, however, be appreciably repaired with old and new technologies. One such new patent-pending technology treats damaged hair with glycidoxy silicone compounds that react with broken cystine bonds and significantly improve fiber elasticity (Syed & Olenick, 2017).

Various older techniques developed over the last 100 years may be used to treat damaged hair. For example, hair fibers may be treated with proteins, where the proteins are trapped inside the hair, thereby imparting marginal improvements in tensile strength. Similarly, treatment with anionic polymers makes the hair feel more bodied and gives the illusion of fiber strengthening. Treatment with anionic polymers does not fulfill consumer needs though for serious, long-term management of hair repair. Over the last decade, keratin and hydrolyzed keratin obtained from sheep's wool are used in combination to increase the elasticity of damaged hair, but since this technology is not a reactive process, it does not permanently repair hair.

Chemists are constantly working to reduce or eliminate the damage from physical processes, chemical treatments, and styling techniques. Although great advances have been made around damage repair, much more needs to be done to achieve truly damage-free hair care products.

## Conditioners for Color-Treated Hair

Conditioners used after permanent coloring or bleaching have several functions such as normalizing the pH of the hair and scalp to 5-5.8, easing wet and dry combing, replenishing the lost moisture of the hair and scalp, strengthening the hair to compensate for lost elasticity, eliminating static electricity, and adding shine to the hair. Therefore, conditioners for color-treated hair should include quaternium compounds to alleviate combing damage, organic acids to normalize the pH of the hair and scalp, moisturizing ingredients, and strengthening agents to recoup lost elasticity and tensile strength.

## Anti-Thinning and Anti-Shedding Conditioners and Serums

Shedding and thinning of hair may be caused by telogen effluvium, requiring medical or alternative treatments. Medical treatments employ Minoxidil as an active in a conditioner-base. Alternative treatments employ combinations of phytosterols, saw palmetto extract, niacinamide, caffeine, fruit extracts, copper polypeptide, and anti-fungal ingredients in the conditioner-base. It is possible to stop the shedding and thinning of hair when these ingredients are used in appropriate concentrations. Hair

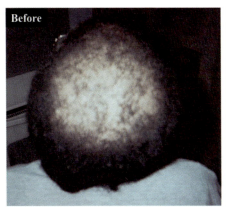 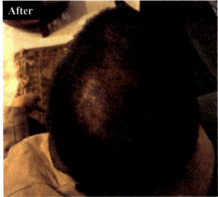

Figure 6.20. Before and after images of a patron who applied an anti-thinning serum containing phytosterols on affected areas of the scalp for 8 months. The after image shows that the vertex of the scalp filled up significantly after treatment.

shedding may stop in two weeks, and an anti-thinning effect could be perceptible in two to six months (see **Figure 6.20**). Anti-shedding results are effective at 50%–60% levels (Syed & Hussain, 2010, p. 22).

Alternative botanical ingredients are added to the base formula of a conditioner composed of gentle quaternium compounds, moisturizing ingredients, organic acids (pH adjusters), anti-fungal ingredients, gentle preservatives, and gentle fragrances. The term gentle fragrance means a fragrance that does not contain endocrine disruptors. This category of conditioners is relatively new in the marketplace, and hair growth performance is low. These conditioners create the perception of hair growth in terms of anti-shedding and anti-thinning to avoid potential conflicts with drug claims.

## Coloring Conditioners

Coloring conditioners contain semi-permanent dyes or temporary dyes in a conditioner base. Temporary dyes or semi-permanent dyes are cationic in nature and compatible with the positively charged quaternium compounds in a conditioner. Here, each formula contains a mixture of dyes that produces a desired shade upon application and rinsing from the hair, such as red, blue, purple, yellow, green, and more. Semi-permanent dyes last on the hair for up to eight shampoos. Temporary dyes last for only one shampoo treatment and allow the consumer not to make a permanent commitment to a particular shade. Temporary dye conditioners also allow the consumer to experiment with various shades before deciding on a permanent hair color.

## Scalp Care While Formulating Conditioners

All conditioning products that touch the hair will also come in contact with the human scalp, no matter how brief the contact time. Therefore, it is essential that all conditioners are capable of balancing the pH of the scalp, moisturizing the scalp, strengthening the stratum corneum, and reducing scalp irritation and inflammation.

## Conclusions

Formulating chemists and hair fiber physicists must familiarize themselves with the various sources and causes of damage to the hair and scalp. Formulation chemists develop products with special ingredients to mitigate damage, whereas hair fiber physicists develop techniques to validate the usefulness of these ingredients and formulations in alleviating or eliminating damage. Measurement of scalp damage and its mitigation is conducted by biotechnologists and formulating chemists with the use of various bioengineering techniques, and selection of appropriate ingredients. The collaboration of these three disciplines is crucial for the development of world-class products.

In this chapter, the various causes of hair and scalp damage were explained in detail. The definitions of various types of conditioning agents were described. Formulation guidelines were provided for a particular type of conditioner for a particular type of damage. Hair chemists and consumers alike must familiarize themselves with conditioners and their specific uses for a given type of damage. Conditioners are a very powerful category of hair care products. They can help resolve many problems associated with hair and scalp damage. If the appropriate conditioner is utilized to treat a specific consumer need, hair and scalp damage can be minimized and even prevented.

## References

Breakspear, S., Smith, J. R., & Luengo, G. (2005). Effect of the covalently linked fatty acid 18-MEA on the nanotribology of hair's outermost surface. *Journal of Structural Biology, 149,* 235–242.

Fair, N.B., & Gupta, B.S. (1987). The chlorine-hair interaction. II. Effect of chlorination at varied pH levels on hair properties. *Journal of the Society of Cosmetic Chemists, 38,* 371-384.

Fair, N.B., & Gupta, B.S. (1988). The chlorine-hair interaction. III. Effect of combining chlorination with cosmetic treatments on hair properties. *Journal of the Society of Cosmetic Chemists, 39,* 93-105.

Garcia, M.L., Epps, J.A., Yare, R.S., & Hunter, L.D. (1978). Normal cuticle wear patterns in human hair. *Journal of the Society of Cosmetic Chemists. 29,* 155-175.

Hoshowski, M.A. (1997). Conditioning of Hair. In D. Johnson (Ed.), *Hair and Hair Care* (pp. 65-104). New York, NY: Marcel Dekker.

Hsuing, D.Y., & Mueller, W. (1979). Hair conditioning waving and straightening compositions and methods. *United States Patent 4,175, 572.* Assignee: Johnson Products, Co., Inc.

Jurczyk, M., Berger, D.R., & Damasco, G.R. (1991). Quaternary ammonium salts. *Cosmetics and Toiletries Magazine, 106*(4): 63-68.

Lotzsch, K.R., Reng, A.K., Gantz, D., & Quack, J.M. (1981). The radiometric technique. explained by the example of adsorption and desorption of 14C labelled Distearyl-Dimethylammonium Chloride on human hair. In Orfanos Montagno & Stuttgen (Ed.) *Hair Research: Status and Future Aspects* (pp. 638-649). Berlin, Germany: Springer-Verlag.

Mettrie, R.D.L., Saint-Leger, D., Loussouarn, G., Garcel, A., Porter, C., & Langaney, A. (2007). Shape variability and classification of human hair: a worldwide approach *Human Biology, 79*(3): 265-281.

Robbins, C. R. (2002). *Chemical and physical behavior of human hair* (4th ed.). New York, NY: Springer.

Robbins, C.R. (1994). *Chemical and physical behavior of Human Hair* (3rd ed.). New York: Springer-Verlag.

Sandhu, S.S, & Robbins, C.R. (1993). A simple and sensitive technique, based on protein loss measurements, to assess surface damage on human hair. *Journal of the Society of Cosmetic Chemists, 44*(2), 163-175.

Syed, A. N. (1986). *Hair softening method and composition.* United States Patent 4,579,131. Assignee: Avlon Industries, Inc.

Syed, A. N., & Gross, K. (1986). *Pre-shampoo normalizer for a hair straightening system.* United States Patent 4,602,648. Assignee: Soft Sheen Products, Inc.

Syed, A. N., Kuhajda, A., Ayoub, H., Ahmad, K., & Frank, E. M. (1995, October). African-American hair: Its physical properties and differences relative to Caucasian hair. *Cosmetics & Toiletries Magazine, 110*, 39–48.

Syed, A. N. (1997). Ethnic Hair Care Products. In Hair and Hair Care. In D. Johnson (Ed.), *Hair and Hair Care* (pp. 235-259). New York, NY: Marcel Dekker.

Syed, A., & Ahmad, K. (1997). Hair strengthening composition and method. *United States Patent 5,639,449*. Assignee: Avlon Industries, Inc.

Syed, A. N. (1997). Ethnic Hair Care Products. In Hair and Hair Care. In D. Johnson (Ed.), *Hair and Hair Care* (pp. 235-259). New York, NY: Marcel Dekker.

Syed, A. N., Ayoub, H., & Kuhajda, A. (1998), Recent advances in treating excessively curly hair. *Cosmetics & Toiletries Magazine, 113*, 47–56.

Syed. A. N., & Ayoub, H. (2002). Correlating Porosity and Tensile Strength of Chemically Modified Hair. *Cosmetics & Toiletries Mag. 117*(11), 57-64.

Syed, A. N. (2006). Hair straightening. In M. Schlossman (Ed.), *The chemistry and manufacture of cosmetics* (Vol. II, pp.535–557). Carol Stream, IL: Allured Publishing.

Syed, A. N., & Hussain, A. (2010). Use of phytosterols anti-shedding and anti-thinning creams or serums. *Avlon Unpublished Research Report 02232010*, 1-29.

Syed, A. N., & Syed, M. N. (2017). *Textured hair: Its characteristics and comparison against non-textured hair. SCC Symposium*, October 12, 2017, New York, NY. 1-31.

Syed, A. N., & Olenick, A.J. (2017). Methods and compositions for treating Damaged Hair. *United States Patent Application No. 2017/013612.*

Syed, A. N., & Olenick, A.J. (2019). Methods and compositions for treating damaged hair. *United States Patent Application No. 16/069,138.* Assignee: Salon Commodities.

# CHAPTER 7

# Hair Styling & Maintenance

After cleansing curly hair with a moisturizing detangling shampoo or a co-wash conditioning cleanser, a deep conditioner is applied to the hair for 15 to 20 minutes and then rinsed out. After a leave-in conditioner is applied, the hair is ready for styling. Thus, hair styling (or setting) is usually the last step in the grooming process, where the hair is set into a desired arrangement, usually with the help of styling aids. Styling products are expected to hold the shape of the style until the next wash.

Formulating chemists must consider the comprehensive needs of curly hair to develop effective styling products for Type 3 and Type 4 hair. For example, styling aids must be easily spreadable on the hair fiber surface, not form flakes on the hair upon drying, should ease combing and manipulation of wet hair, impart slip to the hair, increase moisture, increase shine, and fight humidity in order to avoid reversion and loss of the style or set.

## Types of Styling Products

To accomplish the setting of curly hair, many different types of styling products are available to consumers. These products are as follows:

- Special oil-water sprays
- Twist-defining creams
- Curling jellies
- Curl-enhancing smoothies
- Smoothing gels
- Setting lotions
- Foam setting lotions
- Moisturizing lotions
- Butter creams or curl activators for hair moisturization
- Scalp-moisturizing natural oils
- Edge definers
- Oil sheen sprays

Each of these types of products will be discussed below.

### Special Oil-Water Sprays

This category is new in the marketplace. Oil-water sprays are a unique sub-micron emulsion of natural oils and water. They incorporate hair and scalp renewal additives as well. This author has devised this category to replace the use of ordinary water that is usually sprayed onto the hair during the styling process. These special oil-water sprays enhance the health of both curly and non-curly hair, and are rapidly becoming popular with many different types of consumers.

Two specific examples of oil-water sprays formulated by this author are Jamaican Black Castor Oil (JBCO) Water and Coconut Oil (CO) Water. In these oil-water sprays, the sub-micron emulsion includes an oil phase consisting of each respective natural oil, hair and scalp moisturizers, and hair surface modifiers such as vitamins, ceramides, and phytosterols for strengthening the hair and improving the stratum corneum of the scalp. The use of these "Waters" is intended to replace ordinary water, which is sprayed before and during styling to infuse active ingredients into the hair and scalp, and aid in styling. These oil-waters should be sprayed on the hair if it starts to dry out during styling, which normally may take one hour or more. They may also be used as refreshers for the finished style from Day 3 onward to rejuvenate the style and add extra moisture to the hair.

## Styling Products

Styling products such as twist-defining creams, curling jellies, setting lotions, and foam set lotions are used for setting the hair in a particular style. All of these setting products contain polymers that can impart an effective hold to the hair and keep the style in place. Choosing the type of polymer for an effective hold is very important so that the style will last for a sufficient amount of time (~1-2 weeks). All of these products should contain gentle and safe preservatives whose microbial effectiveness is determined. The consumer trend is away from parabens and formaldehyde-releasers. The fragrance is selected based upon the safety profile with respect to endocrine disruptors (ECDs) and allergens. The next phase of selecting the fragrance is based upon consumer likes and dislikes. Characteristics of each setting product are described in the following sections.

### Twist-Defining Creams

This cream is based on one or more setting polymers such as carbomer, PVP, xanthan gum, pectin, polyquaternium-11, polyquaternium-69, and polyquaternium-55 at a significant level to set hair. This cream also contains 1% to 5% of natural oils, hair and scalp moisturizers, anti-humidity agents, emulsifying agents, fruit extracts for hair strengthening, and hair surface modifiers that mimic the composition of natural lipids in hair. Anti-humidity ingredients are incorporated to fight humidity for a longer hold of the set.

This type of setting cream has a thick texture and lays the wet, wavy/curly hair down smoothly during molding of the hair into a twist shape. Again, JBCO Water or Coconut Water are sprayed during the styling of the hair. Upon drying, the hair is set into many twists all over the head. These twists are taken down into individual strands after 24 hours, when the twists are completely dry. The end result is moisturized, shiny, healthy, and smooth hair strands.

### Curling Jelly

Curling jellies are formulated with mostly natural polymers as setting agents. Some commonly used natural polymers are xanthan gums from beans, starches such as pectin, and gums such as Acacia gum or Gum Arabica. Synthetic polymers can also be added, but the consumer trend leans towards natural or certified organic ingredients. In addition to setting polymers, glycerin is added as a moisturizer along with various plant or fruit extracts as hair strengtheners, natural oils as shine enhancers, and humidity-resistant ingredients. Curling jellies tend to flake from the surface of the hair after drying; therefore, it is important to optimize the level of setting agents in the formulation. The curling jelly is applied to wet hair after a leave-in conditioner; then, the hair is styled using the Wash-and-Go method.

The Wash-and-Go method implies that hair is just stretched and raked into its natural curly pattern with the fingers. The hair is combed, and curls are allowed to form naturally. In some cases, hair is set on curling rods, while keeping the hair soaking wet with Jamaican Black Castor Oil Water or Coconut Oil Water. If the hair is not kept soaking wet at this stage, flakes of the polymers may appear upon drying the hair.

### Curl-Enhancing Smoothie

Curl-enhancing smoothies are cream emulsions that contain hair-setting agents. The cream contains 10% to 15% natural butters (e.g., cocoa butter, shea butter), and natural oils. This mixture of oils and butters is emulsified with the use of hydrophilic emulsifiers, moisturizers/humectants such as glycerin and setting agents similar to the ones used in the twist-defining cream or curling jelly. Before applying the curl-enhancing smoothie, special oil-water sprays (such as a JBCO Water or Coconut Water) are sprayed on wet hair and a leave-in conditioner is applied to the hair. The smoothie is then applied and the hair is styled into twists or any other configuration, while keeping it soaking wet. It is imperative that the hair does not dry out during this styling process. After the styling operation is complete, the hair can be dried under a dryer for 1 to 1 ½ hours. Types 3 and 4 requires almost 24 hours to dry completely. The hair should ideally be air-dried overnight before unfolding. The hair can then be unfolded with the help of a butter cream after a day or two. Incorporating a curl-enhancing smoothie in the styling regime results in a very moisturized and healthy-looking style with enhanced shine.

## Smoothing Gels

Smoothing gels are holding gels for styling the hair. They hold the hair in a given style when applied to wet hair. A number of different holding gels exist, each with a specific secondary function along with the primary function of holding the style in place. For example, holding gels may have secondary attributes of moisturizing, strengthening, or stopping the shedding of hair.

Smoothing or holding gels are formulated with carbomer as a primary hair-holding polymer. Other polymers are added to increase the holding properties for the hair style. These polymers are PVP, polyquaternium-55, polyquaternium-11, and polyquaternium-69. It is important to neutralize carbomer with triethanolamine or aminomethyl propanol first, before adding polyquaternary polymers in the formulation. Usually, a humectant such as glycerin is added to moisturize the hair. For strengthening the hair, hydrolyzed proteins are added. To decrease hair shedding, special proteins such as hydrolyzed lupine protein or hydrolyzed keratin are added.

## Setting Lotions

Setting lotions were very popular in the 1960s and 1970s for setting Type 3 and Type 4 relaxed hair. When blow-drying became popular in the 1980s, hair-setting styles declined significantly. With the resurgence of the natural-hair movement in the 2000s, hair setting became popular again, and thus, setting lotions became relevant again. Setting lotions usually contain water-soluble polymers such as polyquaternium-10, polyquaternium-11, polyvinyl pyrrolidone (PVP), and natural gums, along with glycerin for moisturizing natural Type 3 and Type 4 hair. Other additives include shine- and elasticity-enhancers.

Another type of setting lotion is the foam setting lotion. Here, a small amount of foaming agent is added to the setting lotion formula to create foam during application to hair. Foam setting lotions are packaged with a pump closure that converts the setting lotion into a mousse. Foam setting lotions have become a part of the regimen in styling Type 3 and Type 4 natural hair. Setting lotions and foam setting lotions do not contain significant levels of oils, although some lipophilic moisturizers may be added in the formulations. Many foam setting lotions are clear, water-based solutions, with small quantities of detergents, polymers, and other ingredients.

## Maintenance Products

Products in the maintenance category are moisturizing lotions, butter creams, and scalp moisturizing natural oils. They help maintain moisture and increase the longevity of the style. Hair edge gels are used to define fine hair around the temporal and forehead areas. They are especially useful in holding fine baby hair in a defined form.

### Moisturizing Lotions

Moisturizing lotions are used daily to add moisture and some stylability to the hair. They are oil-in-water emulsions that contain natural oils and butters such as coconut oil, cocoa butter, shea butter, etc., at an approximate level of 25% to 40%. Humectants such as glycerin are included in the formulation to moisturize the hair. As consumers prefer natural ingredients, it is advisable to avoid the use of mineral oil, petrolatum, silicones, parabens, and formaldehyde-releasing preservatives.

### Butter Creams/Curl Activators

As discussed in Chapter 3, Type 3 and Type 4 hair has ~13% to 19% less moisture than Type 1 hair. The primary function of butter creams, which are formulated with natural butters, is to moisturize and retain hair moisture for one to two weeks, that is, until the next wash. They are applied to hair on a daily- or every-three-day basis, depending on the dryness of the hair and scalp. Butter creams contain one or more butters, depending on the properties desired by the consumer. The most commonly used butters are cocoa, shea, mango, cupuacu, illipe, kokum, murumuru, and chia. Illipe butter is used by formulators to increase the stability of the emulsion because of the high melting point of illipe. Murumuru butter is used to impart a silicone-like feel to the emulsion. The addition of certain oils such as castor oil helps to increase the shine of the hair.

Butter creams increase the moisture level of hair and keep it moisturized especially in winter months. Butter cream is applied to dry hair that has already been styled into twisted sections, consisting of subsections of twists/coils. A small amount of butter cream is applied to the fingertips and then applied to the ends of the twisted sections in the hair. Then the sections are unraveled to reveal the coiled/twisted sub-sections. Butter creams also enhance hair shine and can moisturize the scalp directly.

## Scalp-Moisturizing Natural Oils

Natural oils are very popular among consumers with curly hair. These consumers prefer to use natural oils and butters over synthetics like mineral oil and petrolatum. Oils and butters are used by Type 3 and Type 4 hair consumers on an every-three-day basis as a moisture-retaining and anti-drying remedy. These oils and butters are also used on the day of washing the hair with leave-in conditioners and setting jellies or twist creams. Commonly used oils are coconut, olive, argan, Jamaican black castor oil, vitamin E, blackseed, jojoba, monoi, marula, macadamia, almond, avocado, rose hip, and soy. Commonly used butters are coco, shea, and mango.

Tea tree oil is also used on the scalp. It smells like camphor and is extracted from the leaves of the Melaleuca tree; hence, also called melaleuca oil. This oil comes mainly from Australia and is recommended for use against dandruff and acne but limited scientific evidence exists to support these claims. It is not an FDA-approved remedy against dandruff.

Black seed oil comes from the Nigella sativa plant and is found in Asia and the Middle East. It has many health benefits and helps nourish the scalp and hair. It can be taken orally in small doses and is said to build up the immune system. More scientific research needs to be conducted to substantiate such claims.

Neem oil is extracted from fruits and seeds of the neem tree called Azadirachta indica, which is native to the Indian subcontinent; it is cultivated through organic farming and used in medicines and cosmetics. Neem soap is used for skin infections, and neem oil is added to cosmetic products for dandruff control, although no credible scientific evidence exists to that effect. Neem oil is somewhat toxic and cannot be consumed orally.

## Comparing the Moisturization of Oils

The various oils described above were tested for their ability to moisturize hair. The oil samples were obtained from the As I Am® Pure Oils collection. Moisturization was measured using microwave resonance at two different relative humidities: 35% and 70% (results shown in **Figure 7.1** and **Figure 7.2** respectively). The ranking of the moisturizing ability of these pure oils at 35% RH and $p < .05$ was as follows:

**Jamaican black castor oil >**

**Virgin argan oil = Virgin coconut oil = Extra virgin olive oil >**

**Black seed oil >**

**Pure vitamin E oil >**

**Untreated hair**

The ranking of the moisturizing ability of these pure oils at 70% RH and $p < .05$ was as follows:

**Extra virgin coconut oil = Jamaican black castor oil >**

**Virgin argan oil = Extra virgin olive oil = Black seed oil = Pure vitamin E oil >**

**Untreated hair**

All of these oils are moisturizing to hair at 35% and 70% RH when compared to untreated hair, however, Jamaican black castor oil and virgin coconut oil outperformed most of these oils at both summer (75% RH) and winter (35% RH) humidity levels. It is best to use Jamaican black castor oil during the winter and extra virgin coconut oil during the summer.

## Hair Strengthening Comparison of Oils

Most of the tested natural pure oils strengthen the hair. The degree to which each oil increases the elasticity of hair is shown in the graph in **Figure 7.3**. For example, flaxseed oil increased hair elasticity by 10% whereas black seed oil increased hair elasticity by 4%.

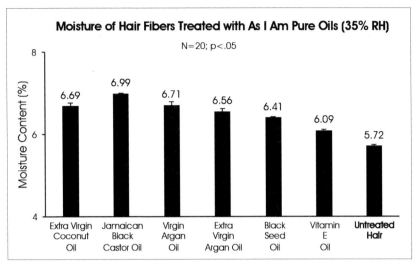

Figure 7.1. Moisture (%) of hair fibers at 35% RH after application of respective As I Am® Pure Oil. Data collected by Avlon® Research Center.

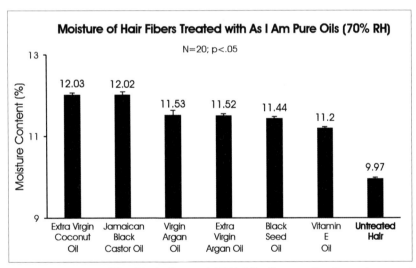

Figure 7.2. Moisture (%) of hair fibers at 70% RH after application of respective As I Am® Pure Oil. Data collected by Avlon® Research Center.

## Hair Edge Defining Gel

It is customary for African-descent consumers to smoothen and flatten the hair around the forehead and temporal areas. Therefore, Type 4 hair consumers generally use stiff and ringing gels to smoothen and lay

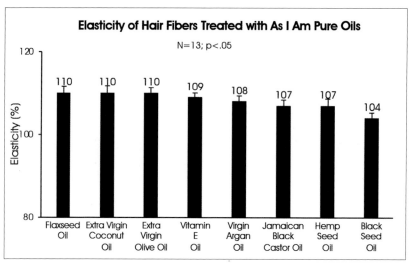

**Figure 7.3.** Elasticity (%) of wet hair fibers after application of respective As I Am® Pure Oil. Data collected by Avlon® Research Center.

baby hair flat on the forehead and temporal area. These gels are called *Hair Edge Defining Gels* and are generally composed of thick microemulsions. They contain very high level of ethoxylated emulsifiers and a small amount of oils for imparting a hold and sleek look to the frontal curly hair. Other additives such as exotic oils and butters are also added for various marketing claims. These emulsions must be formulated carefully because they are clear, or transparent emulsions, and are poured into containers at temperatures as high as 65 to 70°C.

## Oil Sheen Sprays

Oil sheen sprays are used after the hair is styled and dried to provide shine and to alleviate hair and scalp dryness. They are used on a regular basis. Type 3 and Type 4 natural hair consumers prefer not to use mineral oil-based oil sheen sprays. For this reason, a very careful mixture of oils is selected that can be sprayed from a pump. These oils should be low in viscosity in order to form a spray pattern when using the spray pump. Some of the oils of interest are soybean, rice bran, apricot, and grape seed. They can be mixed in high proportions along with some exotic oils such as argan, Jamaican black castor oil, and coconut. This approach to oil sheen spray formulation is based on natural ingredients as opposed to aerosol oil sheen sprays which use propellants and mineral oil. Propellants are now heavily regulated by various governments, especially by the European Union, for safety, human health, and avoidance of environmental pollution. Therefore, the best solution is the use of oil sheen sprays that are based on natural oils.

## Styling Products for Chemically Straightened Hair

Styling products used to style chemically relaxed hair or to straighten hair thermally are discussed in the following sections.

### Blow-Drying Lotions

Blow-drying of wet hair has become very popular among most consumer groups. Thus, after shampooing and conditioning or after any chemical processes, blow-drying is carried out most of the time. In order to avoid excessive repetitive combing damage and thermal damage during blow-drying, blow-drying lotions are sprayed on the hair. These emulsions are liquid in consistency and contain quaternary ammonium compounds, volatile silicones, cationic emulsions of amodimethicones, and fiber-strengthening compounds to help protect the hair against combing and thermal damage (De Marco, Varco & Wolfram, 1985, column 8). Strengthening agents such as fruit extracts, hydrolyzed keratin proteins, and ceramides are also included in these formulations.

### Laminates

Laminates are a newer class of conditioners that were introduced to the market in the mid-1980s. Their use became popular during the early- and mid-1990s. Laminates are based on a combination of various silicones such as volatile silicones, silicone waxes, and dimethicones of low to medium molecular weight. Laminates are very effective in reducing combing damage during repetitive combing or brushing during blow-drying. They also provide reasonable protection against thermal damage (Crudele, Bhatt, Kamis, & Milczarek, 2000, col. 8).

## Anti-Frizz Leave-In Conditioners

Naturally or chemically treated wavy, curly, and coily hair tends to frizz considerably under humid conditions. Frizzing makes the hair unruly and unmanageable. Therefore, there is always a need for leave-in sprays, used as styling aids, to eliminate frizz. The elimination of frizz is an extremely difficult process as most conditioning agents are unable to seal the hair to a degree where the penetration of humidity is completely blocked.

However, emulsions containing volatile silicones and other humidity-blocking compounds help to block the penetration of humid vapors into the hair to a significant level. To illustrate the usefulness and effectiveness of anti-frizz sprays, an experiment was conducted using a commercial anti-frizz spray. The results of the experiment are shown in **Figure 7.4**. Hair tresses were blow-dried and flat ironed with and without the use of a commercial anti-frizz spray. The hair tresses, (1) untreated, (2) treated with a flat-iron, (3) treated with anti-frizz spray and a flat-iron, were exposed to 80% RH in a humidity chamber for 24 hours. **Figure 7.4A** shows the initial condition of the tresses at t=0 hours. **Figure 7.4B** shows the condition of the tresses at t=24 hours, where tress 2 became frizzy and tress 3 remained relatively smooth. Thus, it was apparent that the anti-frizz spray (tress 3) protected the hair most effectively against humidity.

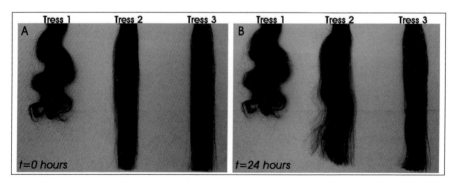

Figure 7.4. Anti-frizz monitoring of three hair tresses at a relative humidity of 80% over 24 hours, where (A) depicts the condition of the tresses at t=0 hours and (B) depicts the condition of the tresses at t=24 hours. Tress 1 was untreated. Tress 2 was treated with a flat iron at 230°C for seven passes. Tress 3 was treated first with a commercial anti-frizz spray and then a flat iron at 230°C for seven passes.

**References**

Crudele, J., Bhatt, D., Kamis, K., & Milczarek, P. (2000). Heat-mediated conditioning from leave-on hair care compositions containing silicone. *United States Patent 6,056,946.* Assignee Helene Curtis, Inc.

De Marco, R., Varco, J., & Wolfram, L. J. (1985). Hair conditioning composition and process. *United States Patent 4,529,586.* Assignee: Clairol Incorporated, New York, NY.

# CHAPTER 8

# Modifying Textured Hair Permanently

Curly hair is often transformed permanently to alter texture, shape, and/or color. Sometimes, temporary treatments may also alter curly hair permanently. It is important to understand how these permanent and semi-permanent processes affect the structure and integrity of curly hair types. Thus, various treatments that alter hair structure permanently, such as relaxing, perming, smoothing, coloring, and lightening will be discussed in this chapter.

Type 4 hair is 23 times more difficult to comb in the wet state and 32 times more difficult to comb in the dry state, as compared to Type 1 hair. Additionally, much more time is required to style textured hair on a daily or weekly basis. Ways to ease the styling process of curly/coily hair are to temporarily thermally straighten, permanently chemically straighten, or permanently chemically wave Type 3 and Type 4 hair. If curly/coily hair is straightened temporarily with the help of heat, it becomes easier to comb and style until the next shampoo. In the past, this process was called *hair pressing*, where an oil-based pomade was applied to the hair, and then a hot metal comb was passed through 3 or 4 times to complete the straightening process (Parks, 1993, p. 14). The metal comb was heated on a stove without any temperature control. This process was very damaging to the hair as it burned the cortex, as shown in Figure 6.2 of Chapter 6. The hair fibers also developed radial cracks, and combing and brushing further accelerated the hair damage, resulting in hair breakage (see Figure 6.3 of Chapter 6). This process has become much safer now where the loss of fiber elasticity is limited to a meager 6% to 8%, thanks to controlled temperatures of blow-dryers and flatirons and especially because of thermal protectants containing volatile silicones.

## Chemical Relaxing

The process of chemical relaxing is defined as permanently transforming curly/coily hair into straight hair. Five types of chemical straighteners can straighten hair permanently: (1) sodium/potassium/lithium hydroxide, (2) guanidine hydroxide, (3) ammonium thioglycolate, (4) sulfites, and (5) smoothing treatments based on formaldehyde/methylene glycol or glyoxylic acid.

Lye relaxers contain alkali metal hydroxides such as sodium hydroxide; no-lye relaxers contain guanidine hydroxide; and no-lye, no-mix relaxers contain lithium hydroxide. No-lye relaxers contain a mixture of calcium hydroxide and guanidine carbonate, which liberates guanidine hydroxide as a straightening agent. While ammonium thioglycolate at a pH of 9 straightens Type 2 and Type 3 hair well, it does not straighten Type 3C and Type 4 hair adequately.

The latest entry to the hair straightening market came from Brazil, in the mid-2000s. These products used formaldehyde gas dissolved in water, also known as methylene glycol, to straighten hair. This category is unsafe for hairstylists and consumers alike because of the potentially carcinogenic nature of the formaldehyde fumes emitted during blow-drying and flat ironing. This category became popular among consumers of Type 2 and Type 3 hair. The advantages of this method are a sleek look and a high resistance to humidity. This category of products has provoked many law suites and regulatory restrictions by the Occupational Safety and Health Administration (OSHA).

An upgrade of this technology came with the use of glyoxylic acid instead of formaldehyde as the active agent. Since glyoxylic acid is a solid material, not a gas, it does not emit the same degree of unsafe and pungent fumes, even during blow-drying and flat ironing. The drawback of glyoxylic acid is its very low pH, where glyoxylic acid systems preclude same day permanent coloring. For example, the consumer must wait a week before permanent hair color application after a glyoxylic acid-based smoothing treatment.

Chemical treatments permanently change the chemical and physical structure of hair fibers and tend to inflict major chemical damage. Chemical damage comes in the form of losing several cuticle layers, fiber elasticity, natural lipids, cuticle CMC, some proteins of the cortex, and moisture of the hair and scalp. Chemical treatments also cause inflammation and irritation of the scalp. The porosity of chemically treated fibers increases, and the hair becomes more sensitive to humid weather and less manageable in hot, humid climates. In low-humidity conditions, the hair becomes dry and brittle. This damage has been mitigated considerably over the last three decades, so that today's relaxers are much less damaging than the relaxers of the past.

## Lye Relaxers

Lye relaxers are based on sodium hydroxide in a cream consisting of water, petrolatum, mineral oil, emulsifiers, and substantive conditioning and moisturizing agents. The cream relaxer is left on Type 3 and Type 4 hair for 13 to 18 minutes and then rinsed off. The pH of the relaxers ranges from 12.75 to 13.25. Mild-strength relaxers contain ~1.9% sodium hydroxide, whereas normal- and resistant-strength relaxers contain ~2.10% and ~2.35% sodium hydroxide, respectively. Alkali metal hydroxide relaxers change one third of the cystine or disulfide bonds to lanthionine bonds, and lead to minor hydrolysis of peptide bonds (Wolfram, 1981, p. 497). The reaction of cystine with sodium hydroxide is shown in **Figure 8.1** (Tolgyesi & Fang, 1981, p. 117).

During relaxing Type 3 and Type 4 hair, the pH of the hair increases and hair swells, which exerts excessive pressure inside the hair. This excessive pressure causes the hair shaft to burst open in the form of longitudinal and radial cracks, as shown in **Figure 8.2**. Additionally, several cuticle layers are lost due to this excessive swelling, as shown in **Figure 8.3**.

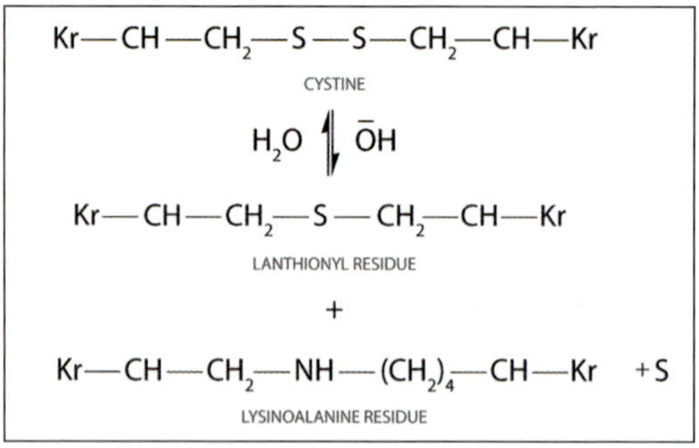

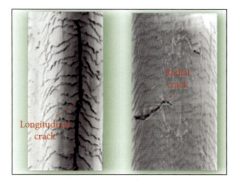

$$Kr-CH-CH_2-S-S-CH_2-CH-Kr$$
CYSTINE

$H_2O \updownarrow \bar{O}H$

$$Kr-CH-CH_2-S-CH_2-CH-Kr$$
LANTHIONYL RESIDUE

+

$$Kr-CH-CH_2-NH-(CH_2)_4-CH-Kr \quad +S$$
LYSINOALANINE RESIDUE

Figure 8.1. Chemical reaction in a kertain hair fiber where one third of the cystine bonds (S-S) change to lanthionine bonds. Kr denotes keratin fiber.

Figure 8.2. Hair fibers develop longitudinal cracks (left) and radial cracks (right) due to increase osmotic pressure during relaxing process. Images obtained using a scanning electron microscope, courtesy of Avlon® Research Center.

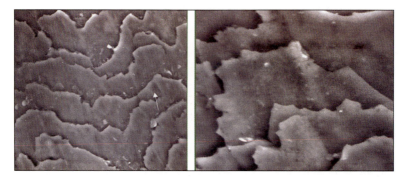

Figure 8.3. The cuticles of untreated hair are not swollen (left), whereas cuticles of relaxed hair (right), are swollen, and some are rinsed away when the relaxer is rinsed from the hair. Images obtained using a scanning electron microscope, courtesy of Avlon® Research Center.

These swollen cuticles deswell when washed with highly acidic normalizing shampoos of pH 5.0. The relaxed hair also loses significant amounts of tensile strength, elasticity, and moisture content. Wet relaxed hair fibers lose as much as 40% of their tensile strength (Syed & Ventura, 2014, p. 2). The loss of tensile strength of dry hair is only 7% for sodium hydroxide (Syed & Milczarek, 2012, p. 2). Relaxed hair also develops excessive static electricity and high porosity. On the positive side, relaxed hair is much easier to comb in both, wet and dry states than untreated Type 3 and Type 4 hair and, thus, less prone to excessive hair loss during combing.

After exposing curly hair to a cream relaxer for 13 to 18 minutes, the relaxer is rinsed from the hair with tepid water. The pH of the hair drops to ~10 when the cream relaxer is rinsed off. The hair is, then, shampooed with a neutralizing shampoo containing commonly used ingredients such as citric acid, mild detergents, and conditioning agents to detangle the hair. The pH of the neutralizing shampoo ranges from 6.0 to 6.5. The hair is, then, conditioned with a special conditioner and styled using the appropriate products.

### No-Lye Relaxers

No-lye relaxers may be more damaging as the hair loses 60% of its elasticity in the wet state and 10% in the dry state. The major advantage of no-lye relaxers over lye relaxers is that they are less irritating to the scalp (Syed & Naqvi, 2000, p. 52). The chemical reaction with cystine bonds is similar to that of lye relaxers. No-lye relaxers contain guanidine hydroxide and straighten the hair more effectively for individuals with a sensitive scalp. They have become an equally important subcategory in the relaxer segment. One major market disadvantage of a no-lye relaxer is that guanidine hydroxide is not stable in the presence of water; therefore, it is prepared in situ by mixing three parts of cream containing calcium hydroxide (5.5%–7.0%) and one part of liquid activator, containing 25% active guanidine carbonate solution in water. The mixture produces guanidine hydroxide, which is an active straightening agent, according to the equation shown in **Figure 8.4**.

This type of relaxer is marketed in three strengths, namely, mild, normal, and resistant, and the pH of these three strengths ranges from

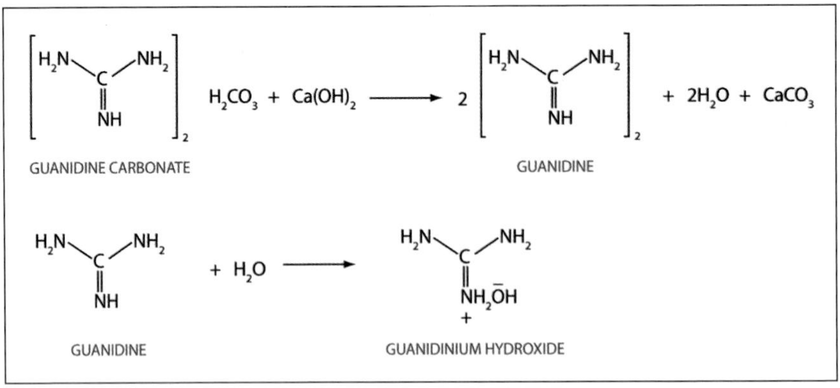

**Figure 8.4.** Chemical reactions showing the liberation of guanidine hydroxide from a combination of calcium hydroxide cream and a solution of guanidine carbonate.

12.75 to 13.25. Like lye relaxers, no-lye relaxers change one third of the cystine bonds of the keratin fiber to lanthionine bonds. However, no-lye relaxers swell the hair significantly more than their lye-counterparts; hence, causing more damage in terms of tensile strength. Wet relaxed hair fibers lose as much as 60% of their tensile strength. Recent advances in no-lye relaxer technology have reduced the swelling of hair by almost half with the addition of deswelling ingredients (Syed & Ahmad, 1994, col. 9), cationic polymers (Syed, 1986, col. 11), and cationic silicones (Syed, 2020, col. 46). Cationic polymers are also responsible for reducing combing damage by making the hair comb more easily in both the wet and dry states. Due to these scientific breakthroughs, this type of relaxer has become considerably less damaging and very popular in the marketplace.

A major disadvantage of this relaxer system is that, once the two components are mixed, any left-over portion after use cannot be saved because the guanidine hydroxide starts to deteriorate into urea and ammonia, which is very damaging to hair. It is important to remember that, once the two components (i.e., the cream relaxer and the liquid activator) are mixed together, they should be used immediately, that is, within 5 minutes, in order to avoid any damage to the hair during relaxing.

### No-Lye No-Mix Relaxers

No-lye no-mix relaxers are based on lithium hydroxide as an active ingredient, while the other ingredients in the relaxer cream are like those of lye relaxers. The reaction of lithium hydroxide with curly/coily hair is also similar to that of lye and no-lye relaxers where one third of the cystine bonds change to lanthionine bonds, leaving two thirds of the cystine bonds intact. Relaxers based on lithium hydroxide are not as effective or efficient in straightening Type 4 hair as sodium hydroxide- or guanidine hydroxide-based relaxers. The manufacturers of relaxers call this category *no-lye no-mix relaxers* and position it as a single component, ready to use and not requiring any mixing with other components. This relaxer system does not enjoy a great deal of success in the marketplace.

**The pH Roller Coaster Before, During, & After Relaxing**

The pH of hair experiences ups and downs during the relaxing process; thus, it is appropriate to discuss this cycle of pH changes and use them for positive outcomes. **Figure 8.5** depicts the roller coaster of these pH changes from before and right after the relaxing process. The pH of untreated healthy hair and scalp is in the range of 5–5.8, and the cuticles of the hair lay flat on the surface of the hair. The pH of cream relaxers is ~13. When this relaxer is applied to the hair, the pH of the hair increases to 13, and the hair starts to swell. It may swell to 50% of its original diameter. The cuticles of the hair are completely open and provide the best opportunity for conditioning. Unfortunately, most conditioners are not stable at a pH of 13. Traditional quaternary ammonium compounds are especially unstable at this high pH. Stable conditioning agents are a few cationic polymers that condition the hair simultaneously as it is being straightened by the relaxer (Hsiung & Mueller, 1979; Syed, 1986). These cationic polymers are able to penetrate deep into the cortex of the hair, strengthening the hair and reducing combing energy as well. Since the molecular weight of these conditioners is large, significant quantities of the polymers remain in the cortex of the hair after rinsing off the relaxer cream with water. These cationic polymers can stay in the cortex of the hair for up to four shampoo treatments (Syed, 2006, p. 557).

After 13 to 18 minutes of relaxer treatment, Type 4 hair becomes straight, and the relaxer cream is rinsed off with tepid water for 4 to 5 minutes. The pH of the hair and scalp drops down to ~10, the hair becomes

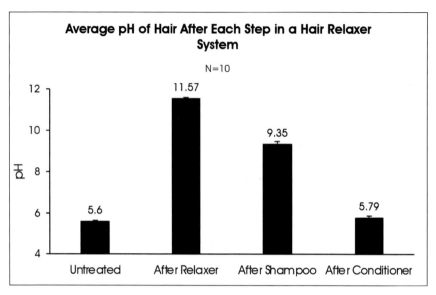

**Figure 8.5.** Graph depicting the pH of the hair at various stages of the relaxing process. Data collected by Avlon® Research Center.

less swollen, and the TEWL value of the scalp is unfavorably elevated. The cuticles are approximately 40% open at this stage. This is the second-best opportunity to condition the hair during the relaxing process. Since the cuticles are partially open, a post-chemical conditioner containing the same cationic polymers and a high dose of organic acids is applied and left on the hair for 5 to 10 minutes. During this treatment, more cationic polymers penetrate the hair cortex and reduce the pH of the hair and scalp from ~10 to ~7.

After rinsing off the post-relaxer conditioner with water, the hair is shampooed with a neutralizing/normalizing shampoo of acidic pH. Generally, a high-quality neutralizing shampoo contains cationic polymers, mild detergents, and organic acids such as citric acid, lactic acid, or acetic acid and hair-strengthening ingredients such as fruit extracts, hydrolyzed proteins, and other strengthening agents.

## TEWL Changes During the Relaxing Process

When relaxers come into contact with the scalp, they increase transepidermal water loss (TEWL) of the stratum corneum. The damaging effects of relaxers upon the scalp can, therefore, be evaluated by measuring

TEWL, moisture, and erythema of the scalp during the relaxing process. The TEWL values of the scalp are shown in **Figure 8.6**.

A conventional sodium hydroxide relaxer was tested on the forearms of 10 participants with an open patch test at 45% RH and 22°C in an environmentally controlled room. All subjects were acclimated to the environment for 20 minutes before the start of the experiment. The baseline of skin TEWL was established first. Then, 0.1 g of relaxer was applied to an area of 7 cm$^2$ on the volar arm site and left on for 10 minutes. After 10 minutes, the relaxer was rinsed off with tap water for 3 minutes, and the skin was blotted dry. Then, the after treatment TEWL readings were taken.

TEWL was significantly higher after the relaxer treatment, as compared to TEWL of untreated skin, $p = .029$. However, TEWL decreased significantly after shampooing, and there was no significant difference between TEWL of untreated skin and skin treated with the relaxer followed by an acidic shampoo at $p = .076$. After 4 hours, TEWL was not significantly different from that of the untreated skin at $p = .095$. Therefore, the TEWL of the stratum corneum is expected to normalize after shampooing away the relaxer. This situation may change, however, depending on the quality of the formulations.

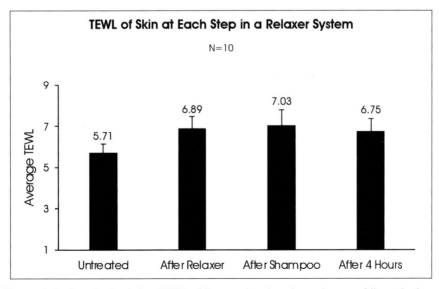

Figure 8.6. Graph depicting TEWL of the scalp at various stages of the relaxing process. Data collected by Avlon® Research Center.

## Deswelling of the Hair During the Relaxer Process

Deswelling agents such as hydrolyzed starches are incorporated in relaxers to help alleviate the erosion of cuticles of the hair fibers, as shown in **Figure 8.7**. The loss of cuticle proteins was measured using the methodology of Sandhu and Robbins (1993, p. 166).

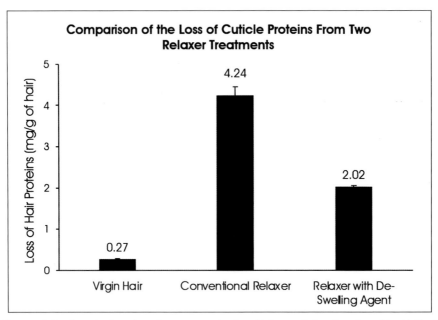

Figure 8.7. Graph showing the amount of cuticle proteins (mg/g of hair) that are lost from the hair after various processes: rinsing (virgin hair), conventional relaxer, and a relaxer with deswelling agent. Data collected by Avlon® Research Center.

In summary, when cationic polymers, deswelling ingredients, and moisturizers are added to relaxer creams, they reduce the loss of elasticity and cuticle proteins, increase ease of wet and dry combing, normalize moisture content, help reduce scalp erythema, and normalize the pH of the scalp (Syed & Kuhajda, 1995, p. 68). The elasticity of wet hair, treated with guanidine, increases from 40% to 80% when these advances in technology are incorporated in relaxer formulations. Similarly, the elasticity of wet hair, treated with sodium hydroxide relaxers, increases from 60% to 85%.

## Smoothing Treatments for Straightening Hair

Most treatments introduced in the marketplace to straighten curly hair under the designation *Brazilian Keratin Treatment* contained formaldehyde as the active material. Only recently have alternative materials such as glyoxylic acid and its derivatives been suggested in this category. Glyoxylic acid, which contains an aldehyde and a carboxylic group, can cross-link with human hair keratin and produce less pungent fumes than formaldehyde. The structure of formaldehyde/methylene glycol, glyoxylic acid, and glyoxylol carbocysteine is shown in **Figure 8.8**.

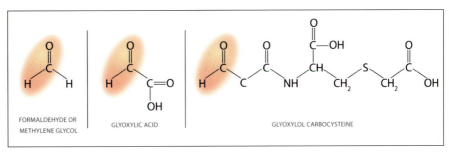

Figure 8.8. The structure of varoius smoothing agents: formaldehyde, glyoxylic acid, and glyoxylol carbocysteine. The aldehyde group is highlighted in each structure.

### Reactions of Formaldehyde with Keratin Fibers

Several types of cross-links can form between the reactive sites on keratin fibers and formaldehyde. For example, the methylene from formaldehyde can insert itself between the two sulfur atoms of cystine to form djenkolic acid ($-S-CH_2-S-$). Some researchers, however, found no evidence of these cross-links. Formaldehyde reacts with both the crystalline and amorphous portions of the keratin fibers. The cystine from both high-sulfur and low-sulfur fractions have equal reactivity with formaldehyde; however, high-sulfur cystine produces carboxylic acid, and the low-sulfur fraction produces djenkolic acid. The point of attack for formaldehyde is at the point of unfolding of the α-helices to form djenkolic acid.

For formaldehyde, cystine is not the only reported site of attack on keratin fibers. Reactions between formaldehyde and the amide and amine groups of keratin are also possible (Hinton, 1974, p. 256). The amine groups can be methylolated, followed by condensation with amide groups. The methylene cross-link is thus introduced as $Kr-NH_2$ (p. 256). Formaldehyde combines with amines and reduces the internal pH of the fiber. Proteins with high concentrations of amides bind large amounts of formaldehyde. It is also mentioned in the literature that two tyrosine moieties in keratin will link via a $-CH_2-$ group of formaldehyde (p. 258). Formaldehyde can cause a cross-link between an amino group of lysine and a peptide group (p. 257). Formaldehyde reacts with the side chains of the amino acids in keratin fibers. For example, side chains of arginine (Arg), lysine (Lys), tyrosine (Tyr), tryptophan (Trp), histidine (His), cysteine, and the amide derivatives of aspartic acid (Asp) and glutamic acid (Glu) can react with formaldehyde (p. 259).

Ziegler (1977) explained that "the primary reaction is the addition of a reactive hydrogen atom to the carbonyl double bond resulting in a methylol derivative. Cross-linking by the methylene group then proceeds via a secondary reaction involving primary amides, guanidyl, and indole groups" (p. 285).

The reactions of glyoxylic acid and glyoxyloyl carbocysteine with keratin are similar to those of formaldehyde, as all three compounds have aldehyde groups that are readily available for cross-linking. However, these two compounds have a much lower pH (0.5–1.0), as compared to formaldehyde (pH≈2.8–4). Thus the pH of systems that contain glyoxylic acid and glyoxylol carbocysteine are normally adjusted to 2.0 with alkali metal hydroxides.

The advantage of these two compounds over formaldehyde is that they do not produce free formaldehyde fumes during blow-drying and flat ironing at high temperatures. Smoothing products containing any of these actives are low viscosity gels or lotions, which are applied to hair after shampooing. They are left on the hair for 30 minutes. The hair is then rinsed lightly with water and blow-dried while enough product remains on the hair. After blow-drying, the hair is flat ironed at 230°C. The flatiron is passed through the hair seven times. The hair becomes very smooth, shiny, and more humidity proof due to the cross-linking of hair keratin with the aldehydic group of the glyoxylic acid or glyoxyloyl carbocysteine.

## Permanent Waving

Humans often desire to change their appearance. If they have straight hair, they want to acquire curly locks, and if they have curly hair, they covet straight hair. Blondes may desire a change to brunette while individuals with black hair may want a softer look towards lighter shades. This human desire for change has created a whole and diverse field comprised of chemists, hairstylists, physicists, biologists, engineers, and dermatologists, all involved in the creation, development, and manufacture of products for human hair, scalp, and skin.

It is this desire to change the appearance of one's hair from time to time that has given rise to the process of permanent waving. Since the development of thioglycolic acid or ammonium thioglycolate, a tremendous body of research has been developed in this area, and the literature displays hundreds of studies on permanent waving of straight hair.

While permanent waving ("perming") was popular among consumers with Type 1 hair for many decades, perms were relatively inconceivable for consumers with Type 4 hair for a long period of time. In 1976, it was Jerry Redding who first started to experiment with permanent waving of Type 4 hair by rolling the hair over toothpicks. This technique created a style that left the hair tightly curled and still looking like an "Afro" of the mid-1950s and '60s. Later, it was Willi Morrow who perfected the art of perming curly/coily hair. His process consisted of first applying an ammonium thioglycolate cream for straightening the hair. In the next step, a Curl Booster lotion containing a small amount of ammonium thioglycolate was applied to the hair. The hair was then wrapped onto perming rods. After 30 minutes, the Curl Booster lotion was rinsed out and the hair was neutralized with a sodium bromate solution. This hair style became popular under the name, *Jerri Curl*. These early perms were very drying to the hair though. Glycerin-based, curl activators became a necessity to combat the dryness and frizziness of permanently waved hair. The permanent-waving process was further improved and maintenance products were introduced, growing the ethnic hair care market tremendously well into the mid-1990s.

This process enabled many women and men for the first time to wear their hair in carefree yet still, curly looking styles.

From the mid-1980s onward, the technique of body perming was introduced, where large rollers were used for wrapping the hair. This technique produced softer, larger, and more fluid curls or waves in curly/coily hair. The term *body perm* originated in the Caucasian market, where it referred to the appearance of thicker hair that provided greater style support. In the ethnic hair care industry, the term was not so much associated with body, or fullness, as with a permanent wave that produced a looser curl pattern, something that had never been achieved with the earlier forms of permanent waving, designed for Type 3C and Type 4 curly/coily hair.

Irrespective of hair type, body perming was for the most part a function of technique where larger diameter rods produced looser curl patterns. Another new technique followed, where long spiral rods were introduced that produced beautiful spiral-shaped curls.

Regardless of the type of rods or rollers used, the chemistry of permanent waving is the same, that is, the hair is reduced with reducing agents such as ammonium thioglycolate or cysteamine and then, rolled onto the desired shape of rods. The chemical reactions of permanent waving are shown in **Figure 8.9**. After 25 or 30 minutes, the hair is rinsed and oxidized

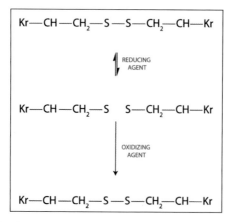

Figure 8.9. Chemical reactions during the perming process. First, the keratin cystine bonds are converted to half cystine (cysteine) when reacted with reducing agents such as ammonium thioglycolate. Next these bonds rebind back to cystine bonds after reacting with oxidizing agents such as hydrogen peroxide or sodium bromate.

with oxidizing agents such as sodium bromate or a mild solution of hydrogen peroxide. The hair is then rinsed again, and the rods are taken out of the hair. This process produces the desired curls or waves in the hair.

During the reduction phase, approximately 20% of the hair's cystine bonds are split into cysteine (or half-cystine bonds). It is during this phase that the hair assumes the new configuration of the rollers. In the oxidation phase, 90% to 95% of the broken cystine bonds are reformed back to cystine bonds to lock in the new curl formations.

The final style of the permanent-waving procedure depends on the selection of the proper rod size for achieving the desired shape: curls, waves, or body. A test curl greatly assists in making an accurate selection of perm rods. As a general guideline, small-diameter rods are used for curls, medium-diameter rods for waves, and large-diameter rods for body perms.

### Changes of pH in Hair and Scalp During and After Perming

The normal pH of the hair and scalp is 5-5.8. During the permanent-waving process, the pH of both the hair and scalp changes, as shown in **Figure 8.10**. The initial pH of the hair and scalp increases to ~9 when

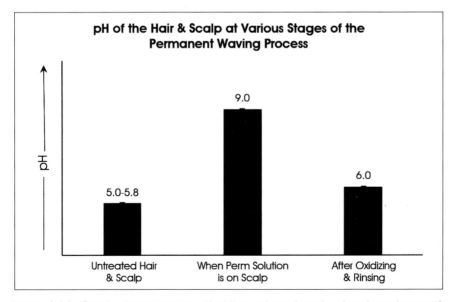

Figure 8.10. Graph depicting the pH of the hair and scalp at various stages of the permanent waving process.

the permanent-waving cream, or curl booster, is applied. After the hair has gone through reduction, it is oxidized with the use of a hydrogen peroxide solution (~2.5% active) for 5 minutes. Since the pH of the oxidizing solution is ~3.5, it can bring the pH of the hair and scalp back to ~6.

### New Method of Perming the Hair

In recent formulations, deswelling agents, cationic polymers, and epoxy silicones were included in permanent-waving creams and curl boosters and solutions (Syed & Olenick, 2020, p. 49). Before perming, the hair was cleansed with a shampoo containing cationic polymers, mild detergents, and acids in order to balance the pH to 5–5.8. The permanent-waving cream should contain deswelling agents and cationic polymers, and the pH should be adjusted to 8.9. The hair is then neutralized. The deswelling agents control the swelling of the hair during perming (also referred to as *reduction*), and the cationic polymers penetrate deep into the cortex to impart more permanent conditioning. Both the deswelling of the hair during perming and inserting cationic polymers into the cortex, strengthen the hair significantly, when compared to the conventional process.

### Straightening Type 2 and Type 3 Hair via Permanent-Waving

Type 2 and Type 3 hair can be straightened with a cream containing ammonium thioglycolate as an active reducing agent. The activity of this cream in terms of thioglycolic acid is ~8%-10%. Rollers are not needed as the hair is being straightened and not waved. When the hair is straight, the cream is rinsed off and neutralized with a cream or lotion containing 2.5% active hydrogen peroxide for 5 minutes. The hair is then rinsed again and blow-dried, using thermal protectants. For the final finish, the hair is flat ironed at 200°C with four or five passes, using thermal protectants containing silicones. This process of hair straightening is popular in the Middle East, South East Asia, Japan, and South America.

## Hair Coloring

The coloring of hair is an old ritual. Its history spans many centuries dating all the way back to the Ancient Egyptian era and continuing into to the Roman, the European, and, finally, to the modern-day era. The chemistry of hair coloring has progressed over the centuries, and the discussion here centers on modern-day hair coloring products.

Hair coloring products fall into three categories: temporary hair coloring, semi-permanent hair coloring, and permanent hair coloring. Recently, marketers have introduced a new category of hair colors, called *hair paints* or *hair makeup*. This category is geared toward consumers who are averse to chemically treating their hair. For example, *naturalistas* with Type 3 and Type 4 hair want to color their hair with non-chemical colorants that will not change the physical or chemical structure of their hair. Therefore, hair paints and hair makeup colors are perfect for these consumers.

### Hair Paint Wax or Hair Makeup

In the category of hair paint wax or hair makeup, pigments are mixed with waxy cream formulations and painted on to the surface of the hair. The hair is then dried, and the color of choice is kept on the hair until the next wash day. These paints completely wash off and do not impart any permanent color change to the hair. The formulations also come in gel form, in addition to waxy creams, with the additional goal of not only painting the hair with pigment but also imparting a nice set in a desired style either by twisting the hair or with the use of the Wash-N-Go technique.

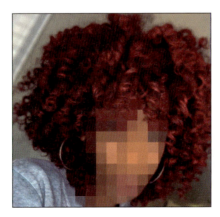

**Figure 8.11.** Red pigmented As I Am® Curl Color was painted on dark-brown hair. Image provided by courtesy of As I Am® brand.

Examples of pigments used in hair paint waxes and hair makeup are iron oxides (CI 77491), ferric ferrocyanide (CI 77510), titanium dioxide (CI 77891), mica (CI 77019), and tin oxide (CI 77861). In addition to pigments, some natural powders of fruits and flowers are added as well. A few Food, Drug, and Cosmetic (FD&C) colors are also blended to acquire a desired shade. However, if FD&C colors are used, they tend to transfer the color to clothes, skin, and hands during application. The advantage of pigments over FD&C colors is that they do not transfer to hair, skin, hands, and clothes significantly. An example of As I Am® Curl Color in a shade of red is shown in **Figure 8.11**.

### Semi-Permanent Hair Coloring

Semi-permanent hair colors can alter natural hair color without hydrogen peroxide, and the effect lasts through six to eight shampoos. Semi-permanent hair colors are based on direct dyes, which are positively charged molecules. Thus, they have an affinity for the negatively charged sites in damaged hair. They are called direct dyes because they are applied to freshly shampooed wet hair, without mixing with developers. Semi-permanent dyes enrich the natural color of the hair. They add shine and tones to the natural color such as gold, red, auburn, purple, blue, and ash. They restore the original shade of graying hair, if the gray hair amounts to less than 30% of the total hair population. They are also able to rid gray hair of its yellowish-green cast. Direct dyes are now very popular among consumers with Type 1 and Type 2 hair. The hair can be treated with direct dyes to give a vivid color of choice such as purple, blue, red, pink, orange, yellow, green, and endless other shades. These shades become more vivid if the hair is lightened prior to the treatment with direct dyes.

Semi-permanent dyes do not chemically react with the hair, as do permanent (oxidative) dyes that require premixing of hydrogen peroxide-based developers. Therefore, semi-permanent colors cannot lift, or lighten, one's natural hair color, nor can they produce a permanent change. Semi-permanent colors are not damaging, unlike permanent (oxidative) dyes. A list of these dyes includes: Basic Blue 99, Basic Red 51, Basic Yellow 87, Basic Brown 16, Basic Brown 17, Basic Orange 31, Basic Red 76, Basic Violet 2, Basic Red 14, and Basic Yellow 40.

## Desired Properties of Semi-Permanent Hair Colors

Among the desired properties of semi-permanent hair colors, expected by professional hairstylists and formulating chemists are the following:

1. Dyes used in the shades must have similar or complementary properties. Approximately 10 independent dyes are used in these shades.

2. The hair has varying degrees of porosity along its length from the root to the ends of hair, but dye take-up must proceed uniformly.

3. The removal of these dyes upon shampooing is very important where all dyes should be removed from the hair at the same rate.

4. All dyes must photo-fade in the same way when exposed to light.

5. All dyes should have the same affinity for the hair since dying time is ideally 30 min but can range from 20 to 45 min.

6. Semi-permanent hair dyes should be simple to use by hairstylists and consumers and offer the highest level of protection from toxicological risks. These dyes should not produce primary irritation of the skin.

7. Coloring should process at room temperature or with the assistance of a heat cap or hooded dryer. Processing time is usually short, from 20 to 30 min. Effective semi-permanent dyes are molecules small enough to adequately penetrate the hair shaft. The molecular structures of such dyes, in fact, have a special affinity for keratin and thus are substantive to the hair.

8. It is important that semi-permanent coloring products do not result in unforeseen hair color changes when they interact with other products such as shampoos, conditioners, and styling products.

9. Reasonable endurance: Semi-permanent hair color should

stand up well to sunlight, atmospheric oxidation, friction, and washing. Stylists and their clients are typically dissatisfied when the color dissipates quickly in sunlight or rubs off on collars and pillows. A good semi-permanent dye retains the same tone, while gradually dissipating throughout the course of six to eight shampoos. At that time, the hair is ready to accept a successive application of semi-permanent color.

### Versatility of Application

A major advantage of semi-permanent hair dyes is that they can be applied to either virgin or chemically treated hair during any given salon visit. Since semi-permanent colors do not change the chemical structure of the hair, they can be applied to the hair after chemical services on the same day. Actually, the hair is even more receptive to semi-permanent colors after relaxing, permanent-waving, or bleaching.

## Hair Lightening/Bleaching

Bleaching/lightening and coloring hair are popular activities for hairstylists and consumers. It is vital that they understand the chemistry of hair lightening. This knowledge is particularly important, given that bleaches and coloring treatments are frequently applied to hair that has been previously treated with relaxers and permanent waves. The lightening of hair is, in fact, the most damaging process of all chemical treatments. While every effort is made to keep lighteners away from the scalp during application, some of the lightening creams end up touching the scalp during the application process of 45 minutes to 1 hour and during rinsing. A lightening cream is a mixture of a high concentration of hydrogen peroxide and a powder lightener. Thus, lightening creams are oxygen donors and can damage the scalp's stratum corneum and even further damage the scalp by causing premature hair loss.

It is important to discuss the chemistry of hair bleaching along with certain technological advances that help keep the hair and scalp in good condition. Bleaching, in a broader sense, is lightening or decolorizing the hair. In scientific terms, it is an oxidation process, carried out at an alkaline pH of ~10, in order to reduce or eliminate the melanin present in the hair. In modern days, this process is employed either to lighten the hair or to prepare hair for the coloring process when a lighter shade than the natural one is preferred. The most common technique is to lighten fibers in small bunches all over the head to give a special effect. The result is hair with a higher tonal level than the natural one. Hair lightening is evaluated on a tonal scale from Level 1, which is black hair, to Level 10, which is the lightest blonde (Zviak, 1986a, p. 215). **Table 8.1** shows the tonal scale from 1 to 10.

Table 8.1. *Natural Tonal Level Scale*

| Color | Scale of Natural Level (N) |
|---|---|
| Lightest blonde | 10N |
| Very light blonde | 9N |
| Light blonde | 8N |
| Medium blonde | 7N |
| Dark blonde | 6N |
| Light brown | 5N |
| Medium brown | 4N |
| Dark brown | 3N |
| Darkest brown | 2N |
| Black | 1N |

Even to this day, all bleaching processes involve oxidation. This process gives lighter shades, resulting in white or blonde hair, depending on the application time and the strength of hydrogen peroxide. The modern-day bleaching process is very damaging to the hair with respect to its loss of strength/elasticity and increase in fiber porosity (Syed & Ayoub, 2002, p. 60). The increase in fiber porosity is associated with hair damage such as a significant loss of elasticity and proteins of the cuticles (p. 62). To change medium brown hair to light blonde, the hair is bleached twice to attain a blonde shade. This bleaching process is termed a double process; it is extremely damaging to hair in terms of its elasticity and tensile strength, moisture loss, porosity, loss of cuticle proteins, cuticle CMC, lipids of the cuticles such as 18-MEA, and split ends.

A considerable volume of literature exists regarding the reactions of hydrogen peroxide and persulfates (powders as accelerators) for decolorizing or lightening/bleaching hair. The bleaching of hair is based on oxidizing the melanin of the hair, which is the natural pigment responsible for hair color. Melanin is produced by a specialized group of cells called melanocytes, by the oxidation of tyrosine and subsequent polymerization. There are three types of melanin: eumelanin, pheomelanin, and neuromelanin. Eumelanin is the most common type; it is usually produced in black and brown hair subtypes. Pheomelanin is a cysteine-derivative, containing red-brown polymers of benzothiazine, which is responsible for red hair and freckles. **Figure 8.12** shows the structure of eumelanin and pheomelanin. Neuromelanin is found in the brain; its function is obscure.

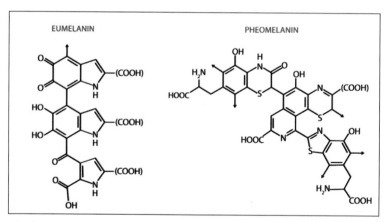

Figure 8.12. Chemical structures of eumelanin and pheomelanin.

## Chemical Damage Due to Lightening/Bleaching

During the process of lightening/bleaching, the melanin pigment, present in the hair cortex, undergoes partial or complete oxidative degradation (Robbins, 2002, p. 155). The oxidizing agents must penetrate the hair structure to reach the melanin in the cortex. Melanin is distributed as ovoid or spherical granules that are between 300 and 400 nm in size (Swift,

1997, p. 56; Wolfram, Hall, & Hui, 1970, p. 880). Therefore, oxidizing agents such as hydrogen peroxide at a pH of 10 must pass through the following components of the hair, before reaching the melanin in the cortex:

- The proteinaceous layer and lipid layer (18-MEA) of the epicuticle
- The A Layer with 35% cystine
- Exocuticles with 15% cystine
- Endocuticles with 3% cystine
- CMC between the sublayers of a cuticle layer
- CMC of the cuticle-cuticle layers
- CMC between innermost cuticle layer and the cortex
- CMC of the cortical cells and the cystine of the matrix
- The peptide- and side-chains of amino acid residues of keratin

During this process, all of the above components of the hair are degraded to some extent, along with melanin. Analysis of the amino acid content of bleached hair showed that cystine, methionine, tyrosine, lysine, and histidine were degraded to the greatest extent (Zahn, Hitlerhaus, & Strubmann 1986, p. 160). It was reported that 15% to 25% of cystine bonds were degraded to cysteic acid in human hair during normal bleaching, and as much as 45% of cystine bonds may cleave during oxidation in the case of frosting (Robbins, 2002, p. 157).

Bleached hair appears drier, more brittle, and rougher to touch. Additionally, bleached hair fibers are difficult to comb, where the combing energy is much higher when compared to that of virgin hair. Elasticity decreases as much as 25% (Syed & Olenick, 2020, p. 41) and porosity increases as much as 75% (Syed & Ayoub, 2002, p. 62). The hair fibers easily split at the ends or along the shaft, as the hair is weakened and not able to withstand the abrasion associated with combing, brushing, and other grooming practices (Robinson, 1976, p. 161).

**Mechanism of Lightening/Bleaching**

Bleaching involves oxidative degradation of disulfide bonds (S-S). It proceeds through S-S fission. It is carried out in an aqueous alkaline oxidizing medium. Two possible mechanisms are mentioned in the literature, and, in each scenario, cysteic acid is produced, and the hair is degraded at various sites (Robbins, 1971, p. 341). The two mechanisms are shown in **Figure 8.13** (S-S fission) and **Figure 8.14** (C-S fission).

S—S FISSION
R—S—S—R
R—SO—S—R
[R—SO₂—SO—R]
R—SO₂—SO₂—R
2 R—SO₃H

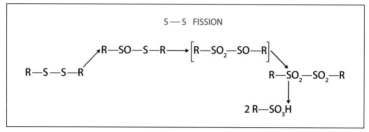

Figure 8.13. Chemical reaction of S-S fission showing the formation of cysteic acid during hair bleaching.

C—S FISSION
R—S—S—R → R—S—S—OH → R—S—SO₂H → R—S—SO₃H → R—SO₃H + H₂SO₄
+
R—OH

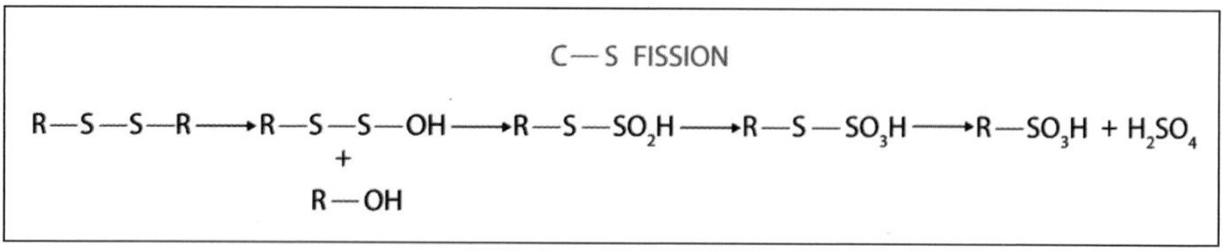

Figure 8.14. Chemical reaction of C-S fission showing the formation of cysteic acid during hair bleaching.

Hydrogen peroxide attacks melanin, solubilizing it, which amounts to ~2% by weight of hair. The pH of the bleaching system is alkaline (between 9.5 and 10.5), and the perhydroxy anion $HO_2^-$ is the reactive species. The attack on keratin is nucleophilic; the cystine linkages are, therefore, very reactive toward oxygen atoms, and the high alkalinity induces disproportionate oxidized species (Wolfram et al., 1970, p. 891). The process also depends on the concentration of $H_2O_2$. There is a linear acceleration in the dissolution rate of melanin upon increasing the concentration of $H_2O_2$. Hence, the higher the concentration of $H_2O_2$, the greater the damage caused to the matrix. When hair is bleached with 3%, 6%, and 9% hydrogen peroxide for 60 to 120 minutes, the cysteic acid content increases by 20%. The cysteic acid content of bleached hair is determined with the use of ion-exchange chromatography and polarography (Erlemann & Beyer, 1972, p. 791) and FTIR spectroscopy (Signori & Lewis, 1997, p. 235).

The lightening of hair is accomplished by applying hydrogen peroxide lotions, mixed with powder lighteners consisting of persulfates. The concentration of hydrogen peroxide lotions could be as high as 9% to 12%. Persulfates of powder lightener are mixed with hydrogen peroxide lotions, known as developers, in order to decolorize darker hair to blonde hair.

The most popular bleaching process uses a powder lightener containing potassium persulfate (61.69%), ammonium persulfate (22. 37%), an alkalizer sodium metasilicate (13.56%), silica as a stabilizer (1.49%), sodium lauryl sulfate as an emulsifier (1.19%), and EDTA as a stabilizer (1.19%). Hydrogen peroxide developers are oil-in-water emulsions with a thin lotion consistency and have the following amounts of hydrogen peroxide in each developer strength:

- 10 Volume developer contains 3.0% hydrogen peroxide.
- 20 Volume developer contains 6.0% hydrogen peroxide.
- 30 Volume developer contains 9.0% hydrogen peroxide.
- 40 Volume developer contains 12.0% hydrogen peroxide.

The most common combination of powder lightener and developer is one part powder lightener to two parts hydrogen peroxide developer. The most preferred developer is 30 volume, in order to avoid excessive damage to the hair structure. The consistency of this combination of developer and powder is like a paste, thin enough for easy application, yet thick enough to avoid any running and dripping onto the face and neck.

## Bleaching and Conditioning Simultaneously

The last decade has seen new advances in bleaching and conditioning that are based on cross-linking technology. The literature on cross-linking technology indicates that efforts were made in the late 1960s and early 1970s, when cross-linking monomers were utilized during the oxidation process. Monomers such as methacrylamide (MAM) and methyl methacrylate (MMA) were polymerized to a high degree of polymerization inside the hair matrix (Robbins, Crawford, McNeil, Nachtigal, & Anzuino, 1974,

p. 407; Wolfram, 1969, p. 550). However, the toxicity profile and safety of these monomers was questionable.

In the 1990s, cationic polymers such as polyquaternium-6 and polymerized cationic amines were applied as pre-conditioners that penetrate the hair matrix and help condition the hair by providing great ease of combing and some increase in elasticity, but not through an internal polymerization mechanism (Sokol, 1975, col. 8; Syed, 1986). Normally, polymers are not able to penetrate the hair fiber because of their high molecular weight; however, during bleaching, the hair cuticles are open due to excessive swelling, so that these polymers are able to penetrate into the cortex. Upon rinsing the hair with water, the hair partially deswells and many cationic polymers with high molecular weight become trapped inside the cortex. Additionally, some of these high molecular weight cationic polymers ionically bond to the negative sites on the surface of the hair. Polyquaternium-6 makes the hair comb very easily in both the wet and dry states, thereby minimizing combing damage.

In 2016, a new system of polymerization during bleaching was introduced. Here, monomers, two molecules of maleic acid attached with a linker, were applied to the hair during bleaching and coloring, and supposedly polymerized inside the hair, leaving hair strengthened after the treatment (Pressly & Hawker, 2017, col. 23). The structure of this monomer is shown in **Figure 8.15**. Elasticity data was not presented by the inventors; rather, qualitative inferences were presented, based on the feel and look of the tresses.

A new and effective technology was introduced in 2017, where oli-

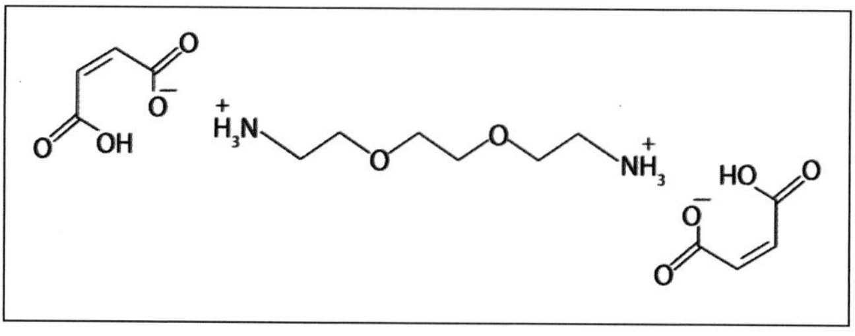

Figure 8.15. The structure of two molecules of maleic anyhydride attached through a linker. These molecules are used for polymerization of bleached hair and color-treated hair.

gopolymers based on epoxysilicones were mixed with the bleaching treatment and left on the hair for 50 minutes. The hair was then rinsed and shampooed with a non-conditioning shampoo. The elasticity of the hair bleached without epoxysilicones was 74%; when epoxysilicones were added, the elasticity of the bleached hair increased to 99%. Furthermore, hair breakage decreased significantly during repeated combing and brushing (Syed & Olenick, 2020, p. 41). The structure of an epoxysilicone is shown in **Figure 8.16**.

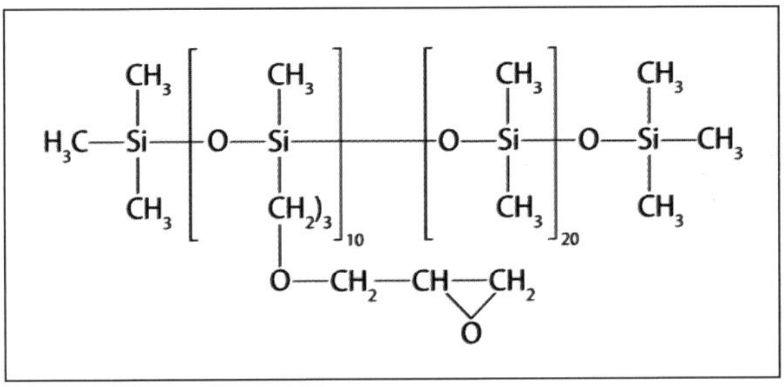

Figure 8.16. The structure of an epoxy silicone oligomer which polymerizes within the keratin fiber during bleaching, coloring, relaxing, and permanent waving.

Bleaching should always be approached with extreme caution, and a strand test should always be conducted first. Bleaching should not be conducted on relaxed African-descent hair, as this hair has elevated porosity and low tensile strength as a result of chemical treatment.

## Permanent Hair Coloring

Permanent dyes are based on oxidative dyes that are mixed with hydrogen peroxide to impart permanent color to the hair that could last for up to 24 shampoos. Permanent dyes are the dominant segment within the hair color market and are the most frequently used product throughout the world. Market growth of this category is significantly greater than for other categories in the hair care market. Today, bleaching and hair coloring continue to be widely used by women and increasingly by men as well.

Permanent hair colors offer the possibility of covering gray or white hair completely and in many shades of personal liking, while simultaneously lifting the natural pigment and depositing artificial color. An array of choices lets consumers select the shades of their liking. These colors or shades are enduring and require only periodic new-growth touch-ups, usually every four to six weeks.

Most of the time, the oxidative dye compound is colorless or has a mere tinge of color. Permanent hair color evolves when an oxidative hair dye in a particular shade is mixed with a developer containing hydrogen peroxide, thereby producing intermediate coloring compounds. These intermediate coloring compounds are responsible for coloring the hair permanently.

Permanent hair colors or dyes are divided into three major chemical families: aromatic para-diamines, para-aminophenols (or amino naphthols), and phenols (or naphthols). The development and manufacture of high-quality, oxidative (permanent) hair color requires ample experience and several practical trials on hair of all types, textures, and degrees of gray.

## Basic Theory of Mixing Colors

Most colors and shades are derived from just three basic colors: red, blue, and yellow. These pigments are known as *primary colors* because they cannot be made by mixing any other colors. When equal amounts of primary colors are mixed, the resulting colors are considered to be secondary colors. The *secondary colors* are violet, orange, and green. *Tertiary colors* are made by mixing equal amounts of primary colors (red, blue, or yellow) with their immediately adjacent secondary colors. In this way, six new combination colors are produced, which are third-level or tertiary colors. The tertiary colors are red-violet, red-orange, blue-violet, blue-green, yellow-orange, and yellow-green.

## The Color Wheel

The color wheel is formed by the systematic placement of primary, secondary, and tertiary colors in a circle. It is quite useful in helping to organize one's thought processes in the basic theory of mixing colors. Ideally, the center of the color wheel is black; black color is produced when all three primary colors are mixed in equal amounts. However, if these primary colors are mixed in unequal amounts, they will produce brown. The shade of brown will vary, depending on the proportions of primary colors used. For example, more red color will create a reddish-brown shade, more yellow will produce golden brown, and more blue will produce a cool brown tone.

Colors positioned opposite each other on the wheel are called *complementary colors*. These opposite complementary colors produce neutral shades of brown (e.g., red and green, when mixed in equal amounts, produce neutral cool brown). The same is true for yellow and violet, which are opposites on the color wheel. The color wheel is shown in **Figure 8.17**.

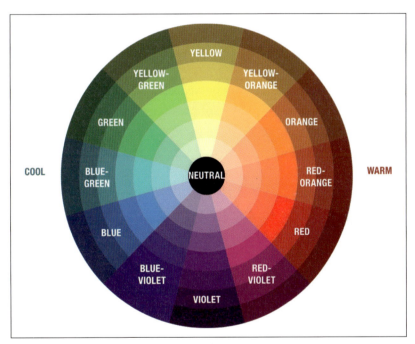

Figure 8.17. The color wheel showing primary, secondary, and tertiary colors along with cool and warm shades. Image provided by courtesy of Avlon® Research Center.

## The Significance of the Color Wheel

The color wheel can be used as a guide for color neutralizing or modifying the tonality of the hair. From time to time, it is necessary to adjust colors that have produced undesirable effects or results. For example, if a green-based color is too green, by utilizing the color wheel, the colorist can add a small amount of red base to correct the problem. Similarly, if a yellow-based color has produced too much yellow in the hair, a violet base (opposite to yellow on the color wheel) can be added to neutralize yellow and attain the desired result.

## Modifying Tonality

The tone of a hair color is what we see reflected as highlights. Hair can either have warm, cool, or neutral tones. Tones can be enhanced or diminished by the addition of colors selected from the color wheel. To enhance a red tone, yellow can be added to warm up the red. To diminish a red tone, violet can be added, which cools down the red. Thus, modifying the color tone of hair affects the highlights of the hair.

## Color Properties of Hair

The natural color of the hair depends on the presence of natural pigments called *melanin*. The color of hair varies not only from one individual to another, but also within the same individual and, sometimes, on different spots of the same hair fiber. It is an accepted fact that all varieties of hair color are derived from two different natural pigments: blue-black and red-yellow. The quantity of these pigments, their distribution inside the hair shaft, and their chemical characteristics determine the color of each hair fiber.

**Depth of color.** The cortex of the hair contains granular melanin, which may be concentrated or diffused. Dark hair contains more concentrated granular pigment; therefore, it has greater depth of color. Blonde or red hair has more diffused pigment (i.e., more spread-out, less concentrated melanin), which gives it less depth of color. The term depth of color, thus, refers to the lightness or darkness of a hair color.

**Hair tone.** All hair colors have tone. Tone is simply the highlights one sees in the hair color. Tone can be warm (red or gold) or cool (absence of red or gold). The depth of color is just how light or dark the hair color is. The human eye is able to distinguish about 10 natural hair colors, which are measured in levels and assigned a number, as shown in **Table 8.1**.

With respect to tone, hair with more yellow-red pigment is de-

Curly Hair: Structure, Properties, & Care  Chapter 8

scribed as warm. Hair that has less of this pigment is considered cool. A person can have hair that is dark and warm—meaning, dark for depth and warm for tone—or conversely, hair that is light and cool—light in depth and cool in tone.

Some pertinent facts to know regarding hair color are that dark hair is more dominant than light hair as a hereditary trait; that gray hair is produced by a partial or total absence of melanin; and that graying is not always due to aging, but can be the result of genetics or a serious illness. When returning gray hair to its original color, the stylist must consider the client's skin tone in order to select an appropriate shade. Most permanent colors come in two parts: Part 1 is in the form of a gel or cream, and Part 2 is a hydrogen peroxide solution or emulsion, ranging from 5-volume (for more color deposit) to 40-volume (for more lift).

**Gel colors.** Gel colors have an oily appearance and are packaged in dispenser bottles. When mixed with hydrogen peroxide developers (usually weight for weight), a clear gel is formed and then applied to the hair. The developer contains a thickening agent, which helps to thicken the mixture of Part 1 and Part 2. Gel colors are very popular because application can be confined to a certain portion of the hair without the danger of running onto previously colored portions of the hair shaft. They are easy to measure and apply, and being transparent, the color development on the hair can be seen without difficulty. Gel colors contain soap type thickeners, derived from fatty acids such as oleic acid, and are, therefore, drying to African-descent hair.

**Cream colors.** Cream colors have become increasingly popular because they offer a number of advantages over gel type colors. Being non-liquid, cream colors are easily applied to the hair fiber. They remain on specific areas, lessening the chance of running onto previously colored hair. They are often formulated with emollients and detangling ingredients, which provide better conditioning. The product consistency has a relatively high level of stability when packaged in a tube container, which decreases product spoilage and enhances performance consistency. Cream colors leave a softer feel to African-descent hair, compared to other types of permanent colors.

## The Action of Permanent Hair Colors on the Hair

Permanent hair colors work in a pH range of 10 to 11. This range is achieved by mixing an ammonia-based cream color (Part 1) with a hydrogen peroxide-based developer (Part 2). The two processes of lifting natural pigment from the hair and depositing artificial pigment occur simultaneously. The objective, when formulating a permanent color, is to achieve a precise balance between the concentration and nature of the dye precursors and the ammonia content; this is directly related to the lifting power of the color formula. It is a very painstaking process for an R&D chemist to formulate a high-quality lifting-and-depositing formula. Many trials are required to optimize the formula.

The two processes of lifting and depositing take place simultaneously, where the lifting of the natural color is the same for all shades, but the depositing of dyes varies from shade to shade. For example, the black (1N) shade lifts to the same degree as a blonde shade. However, the black color (1N) contains high concentrations of brown dyes and, thus, deposits a great deal of the dyes back into the hair, whereas a blonde shade consists of very low concentrations of dyes and, consequently, a small amount of dye is deposited. It appears to the eye that the black color did not lift, when, in reality, it has lifted. By mixing the color cream with varying volumes of hydrogen peroxide (i.e., the developer), different color results can be achieved.

The alkaline pH of the color mixture swells the hair fiber mildly and raises the cuticles, allowing the small dye precursor molecules to penetrate the cortex. The longer the color cream remains on the hair, the larger the dye molecules become through oxidation. After processing, the dye molecules have become so large that they cannot escape the hair shaft, and the artificial color stays permanently inside the hair fiber.

The coloring results are more suitable when the natural hair color is not lifted more than two levels. The final result (or color achieved) is determined by the natural color of the hair prior to color treatment; the artificial hair color selected; the volume of hydrogen peroxide used for processing; processing time; and conditioning of the hair before and during coloring.

Some permanent hair colors are known to deposit color without lifting the natural hair pigment. This is due to the absence of ammonia in the tint formulation. Permanent hair colors of this kind can be used when the colorist desires to match the natural hair color or achieve a darker shade permanently.

### Mechanism of Single- & Double-Process Permanent Hair Color

Permanent hair coloring is a very popular way of coloring hair. One must be careful in selecting the right color for the client through expert analysis and consultation. There are two basic methods of applying permanent hair color: single-process coloring and double-process coloring.

**Single-process permanent coloring.** Single-process permanent coloring is completed in one application, as the name implies. Products in this class contain a lightening ingredient (hydrogen peroxide) as the developer that starts lightening the hair, while the color cream ingredients start the coloring process. The coloring molecules are small enough to penetrate through the cuticle layers into the cortex and, then, are oxidized and augmented in size to form active intermediate molecules by hydrogen peroxide. The active intermediates react with the color couplers that have already been added to the color cream formula. It is the intermediate color molecules and the color couplers that react to provide shampoo-resistant hair dyes. Simultaneously, some of the lightening action is carried out by the hydrogen peroxide (i.e., the developer) present in the product mixture; however, much less oxidation of cystine of the keratin takes place, when compared to double-process coloring. Here, the damage is minimized because, during the formation of active intermediates, the coloring molecules join in to consume most of the hydrogen peroxide, leaving little hydrogen peroxide to break cystine bonds of keratin fibers, which can be considered a fortunate situation.

**Double-process permanent coloring.** Double-process coloring is completed in two applications. First, the hair is lightened to the degree necessary; then, a desired toner is applied. Here, even dark hair can be transformed into a delicate shade of blonde. The lightening of hair is a severely damaging process for keratin fibers; 10% to 20% of cystine is lost during lightening (Wolfram, 1981, p. 495). The decrease in cystine content is matched by the increase in cysteic acid, the undesirable end product of bond breakage.

Some scientific studies indicate that hair undergoes excessive swelling in the double-process coloring method. Apart from swelling, the presence of cysteic acid residues affects the chemical reactivity of hair when it is further chemically treated with permanent waving and relaxers. Therefore, one should use double-process coloring as a last resort. In particular, permanent waving or permanent straightening should not be performed. The application instructions provided by the manufacturer should be closely followed when applying permanent hair color.

## Conditioning During Permanent Coloring

Great advances have been made with respect to alleviating hair damage during permanent hair coloring by using cross-linking monomers or oligomers. The addition of oligomers such as epoxysilicone have reduced the damage to tensile strength to the point of being almost negligible. In multiple experiments, when hair was treated with 6RR dye formula, the elasticity of hair fibers decreased to 88%. The same 6RR dye formula, containing epoxysilicone, left 99% of the elasticity intact. The loss of fiber elasticity before and after treatment was not significant ($p = .346$, which is $> .05$) (Syed & Olenick, 2020, p. 54).

## Conditioning During Double-Process Color Application

The damage to hair fibers with a double process is extensive, as noted in connection with the hair lightening/bleaching process. During hair lightening, the loss of fiber elasticity is ~25%, but with the addition of epoxysilicone oligomers, the damage is reduced to almost zero. In some cases, when epoxysilicone and catalysts were used during and after bleaching, the result was zero loss of hair elasticity, and thus, no significant difference in fiber elasticity before and after treatment ($p = .42$, which is $> .05$) (Syed & Olenick, 2020, p. 41). The damage during toning with a submicron emulsion of epoxysilicone is not significant with this cross-linking technology.

## References

Erlemann, G. A., & Beyer, H. (1972). Die Alkalilöeslichkeit Als Kriterium Für Chemische Und Physikalische Veränderungen Am Humanhaar (Alkali solubility – a criterion of changes in the physical and chemical properties of human hair - Translation). *Journal of the Society of Cosmetic Chemists, 23*, 791-802.

Hinton, E. H. (1974). A survey and critique of the literature on crosslinking agents and mechanisms as related to wool keratin. *Textile Research Journal, 44* (4), 233-292.

Hsiung, D.Y., & Mueller, W.H. (1979). Hair conditioning, waving and straightening compositions and methods. *United States Patent No. 4,175,572*. Assignee: Johnson Products Co. Inc.

Parks, C. (1993). Living Legends in Cosmetology. *Shop Talk, 12*(1), 14-17.

Pressly, E. D., & Hawker, C. J. (2017). Kertin treatment formulations and methods. *United States Patent No. 9,668,954*. Assignee: Liqwd, Inc.

Robbins, C. R. (1971). Chemical aspects of bleaching human hair. *Journal of the Society of Cosmetic Chemists, 22*, 339-348.

Robbins, C. R. (2002). *Chemical and physical behavior of human hair* (4th ed.). New York, NY: Springer.

Robbins, C. R., Crawford, R., McNeil. D. W., Nachtigal, J., & Anzuino, G. (1974). Polymerization into human hair. *Journal of the Society of Cosmetic Chemists, 25*, 407–421.

Robinson, V. N. E. (1976). A study of damaged hair. *Journal of the Society of Cosmetic Chemists, 27*, 155–161.

Sandhu, S. S, & Robbins, C. R. (1993). A simple and sensitive technique, based on protein loss measurements, to assess surface damage on human hair. *Journal of the Society of Cosmetic Chemists, 44*(2), 163–175.

Signori, V., & Lewis, D. M. (1997). FTIR analysis of cysteic acid and cysteine-s-thiosulphate on untreated and bleached human hair. *Macromol Symposium, 119*, 235–240.

Swift, A. J. (1997). *Fundamentals of human hair science*. Weymouth, England: Micelle Press.

Syed, A. N. (1986). Hair softening method and composition. *United States Patent No. 4,579,131*. Assignee: Ali N. Syed, Hazel Crest, IL.

Syed, A. N. (1997). Ethnic hair care products. In D. Johnson (Ed.), *Hair and Hair Care* (pp. 235–259). New York, NY: Marcel Dekker.

Syed, A. N. (2006). Hair straightening. In M. Schlossman (Ed.), *The chemistry and manufacture of cosmetics* (Vol. II, pp. 535–557). Carol Stream, IL: Allured Publishing.

Syed, A. N. (2020). Hair relaxer compositions and method. *United States Patent No. 10,568,829*.

Assignee: Avlon Industries, Inc.

Syed, A. N., & Ahmad, K. (1994). Composition and process for decreasing hair fiber swelling. *United States Patent No. 5,348,737*. Assignee: Avlon Industries, Inc.

Syed, A. N., & Ayoub, H. (2002). Correlating porosity and tensile strength of chemically modified hair. *Cosmetics & Toiletries Magazine, 117*(11), 57-64.

Syed, A. N., & Gross, K. (1986). Preshampoo normalizer for a hair straightening system. *United States Patent No. 4,602,648*. Assigned to Soft Sheen Products, Inc.

Syed, A. N., & Kuhajda, A. (1995). The loss of protein in hair from the treatment of relaxers. *Avlon Research Center*. Unpublished Report No. FN 141, 68–72.

Syed, A. N., & Milczarek, P. (2012). Elasticity of hair at various humidities when treated with guanidine relaxer and sodium hydroxide relaxer. *Avlon Research Center*. Unpublished Report No. 2012-7-27, 1–6.

Syed, A. N., & Naqvi, A. R. (2000). Comparing the irritation potential of lye and no-lye relaxers. *Cosmetics and Toiletries Magazine, 115*(2), 47–52.

Syed, A. N., & Olenick, A. J. (2020). Methods and compositions for treating damaged hair. *European Patent No. 3,402,575*. Assignee: Salon Commodities.

Syed, A. N., & Ventura, T. (2014). The effect of hair relaxers on the elasticity of hair. *Avlon Research Center*. Unpublished Report No. 14–31, 1–4.

Wolfram, L. J. (1969). Modification of hair by internal deposition of polymers. *Journal of the Society of Cosmetic Chemists, 20*, 539–553. Wolfram, L. J., & Albrecht, L. (1987). Chemical and photobleaching of brown and red hair. *Journal of the Society of Cosmetic Chemists, 82*, 179–191.

Wolfram, L. J., Hall, K., & Hui, I. (1970). The mechanism of hair bleaching. *Journal of the Society of Cosmetic Chemist, 21*, 875–900.

Wolfram, L.J. (1981). The reactivity of human hair: A review. In Orfanos, Montagna, & Stuttgen (Eds.), *Hair research: Status and future aspects* (pp. 479–500). Berlin, Germany: Springer.

Zahn, H., Hitlerhaus, S., & Strubmann (1986, May/June). Bleaching and permanent waving aspects of hair research. *Journal of the Society of Cosmetic Chemists, 37*, 159–175.

Ziegler, K. (1977). Crosslinking and self-crosslinking in keratin fibers. In R.S. Asquith (Ed.). *Chemistry of natural protein fibers* (pp. 267–296). New York, NY. Plenum.

Zviak, C. (1986a). Hair bleaching. In C. Zaviak (Ed.). *The science of hair care* (pp. 213–233). New York, NY: Marcel Dekker.

Zviak, C. (1986b). Hair coloring: Nonoxidation coloring. In C. Zaviak (Ed.). *The science of hair care* (pp. 234–261). New York, NY: Marcel Dekker.

# Index

## A

A Layer  13, 27
Alopecia areata (AA)  74
Aloe vera  87, 93
Amino acids  27, 93
Amino acids and proteins  90
Anagen  67, 94
Androgens  94
Androgenetic/androgenic alopecia (AGA)  71, 94
Angstrom  27
Antioxidants  95
Arrector pilli muscles  65, 95

## B

Basal layer  95
Beta-sitosterol  86, 96
Biotin  86, 96
Blood vessels  96

## C

Capillaries  96
Catagen  96
Causes of hair and scalp damage  162
    Chemical treatment-  167
    Chlorinated water-  166
    Combing and brushing-  163
    Shampooing-  162
    Thermal-  164
    Weather related-  164
Causes of hair loss  71
    Alopecia areata (AA)  74
    Androgenetic/androgenic alopecia (AGA)  71
    Central centrifugal cicatrical alopecia  75
    Chemically induced alopecia  75, 97
    Diet deficiencies or overload  79
    Menopause  79
    Seborrheic dermatitis/dandruff  76
    Traction alopecia  73
Cell membrane complex (CMC)  8, 11, 27
    Types of-  11
Cell differentiation  97
Cell proliferation  97
Chemical relaxing  210
    Deswelling during relaxing  218
    Lye relaxer  211
    No-lye relaxers  213
    No-lye no-mix relaxers  214
    pH roller coaster  215
    Reactions of formaldehyde  219
    Smoothing treatment  219
    TEWL changes during relaxing  216
Classes of quaternary compounds  168
    Aminofunctional silicones  174
    Dialkyl quaternary compounds  170

Diester quats   172
Dimethicones   173
Ester quats   171
Homo- and copolymers   174
Monoalkyl quaternary compounds   169
Combing   42
Combing of Type 3 and Type 4 hair   42
   Ease of dry combing   43
   Ease of wet combing   43
Copper deficiency   97
Cortex   8, 15
Cortical cells and hair shape   16, 17, 18
Cortical cells   11, 15
   Para- and ortho-   15, 18, 20
Cross-section of hair   27
Curl activators   200
Cuticles   8
   Architecture   8
   Cuticle layers   10, 12
   Loss of-   134

## D

Density of hair   54
Detergents   116
   Anionic   116
   Amphoteric   122
   Cationic   126
   Classification   116
   Effect on hair   111, 132
   Effect on skin   112, 134
   Natural detergents   128
   Nonionic   126
Dermal papilla   62, 97
Diet difficiencies or overload   79
Differences in Caucasian and African-descent hair and scalp   110

Dimers  8, 26

## E

Elasticity  28
Elasticity, wet  45
Elastic region  28
Elasticity comparison  45
Ellipticity  19, 28, 42, 46
Ellipticity variance  43
Epithelial tissue  97
Endocuticles  14, 29
Epicuticle  12, 29
Exocuticles  14, 29
Exogen  68, 97
External lipids of hair  29

## F

Factors influencing penetration of conditioners  178
    Heat  180
    Length of treatment time  179
    pH  181
Fatty acid  88
F Layer  11, 12
Folic acid  90
Follicle  62, 65

## G

Glycine  29, 120
Growth rate of hair  43, 53, 54
    Comparison of-  69

## H

Hair bulb   63, 97
Hair coloring   224
    Bleaching/conditioning simultaneously   233
    Chemical damage due to lightening   230
    Hair lightening   228
    Hair paint wax or make up   225
    Mechanism of hair lightening   231
    Semi-permanent hair coloring   226
Hair follicle   62
    Arrector pili muscles   65
    Bulb   63
    Dermal papilla   62
Hair & scalp cleansing practices   110
    Effect on hair   132
    Effect on skin   134
    Loss of cuticle proteins during shampooing and wet combing   134
    Moisture content and surface lipids   133
    pH   133
    Physics of cleansing   131
    Prior to shampooing   130
Hair bulb and shape of textured hair   65
Hair follicle matrix   97
Hair growth   66
Hair growth cycle   67-69
Hair growth comparison – Caucasian vs African   69
Hair growth-Lewallen study   70
Hair growth-Loussouarn study   69
Hair loss   71
Hair loss treatments   80
Hair loss remedies   80
    Alternative botanical treatments   85
    Medical treatments   81
    Natural ingredients as additives   85
        Aloe vera gel   87
        Amino acids and proteins   90
        Biotin   86

    Copper   86
    Fatty acids   88
    Folic acid   90
    Green tea   86
    Iron   88
    Niacin   88
    Selenium   89
    Vitamin A, D and E   89
    Zinc   88
  Surgical hair transplants   91
Hair matrix   64, 97
Hair styling and maintenance   195
Hair transplant   91, 98
Heterodimers   29
Hydrogen bonding   29
Hydrophilic   29
Hydrophilic sulfur rich protein   29
Hydrophobic   30
Hypertrichosis   81, 98

# I

Impact of detergents on hair & scalp integrity   111
Inner root sheath (IRS)   64
Intermacrofibrilar matrix   8, 21, 30
Intermediate filaments   8, 21, 30
Internal lipids of hair   30
Iron deficiency   88

# K

Keratin fiber   30

# M

Macrofibrils   21, 30

Maintenance products   200
    Butter creams   200
    Hair edge defining gels   203
    Moisturizing lotions   200
    Oil sheen sprays   204
    Scalp moisturizing natural oils   201
Matrix   22, 30
Medulla   8, 26, 31
Microfibrils   21, 31
Micron   31
Mitigating deleterious effects of sodium lauryl sulfate on skin   114
Mitigation of hair damage using conditioners   168
Moisture of hair   56, 133
Moisture measurement of scalp   98
Methyleicosanoic acid (18-MEA)   12

# N

Nanometer   31

# O

Orthocortical cells   15, 31
    Arrangement in Type 4 hair   24
Outer root sheath (ORS)   64, 98

# P

Paracortical cells   15, 31
    Arrangement in Type 1 hair   24
Peptide   31
Permanent hair coloring   235
    Action of permanent color on hair   240
    Basic theory of mixing colors   236
    Color properties of hair   238
    Conditioning during permanent coloring   242

Condition during double process coloring  242
Cream colors  239
Gel colors  239
Mechanism of single and double process  241
The color wheel  236
Significance of color wheel  237
Permanent waving  221
    pH changes in hair and scalp  223
    New method of perming hair  224
    Straightening hair  224
Polypeptide  31
Porosity  50
Porosity comparison  53
Protein  31
Product development process  137
Protofibrils  24, 31
Protofilaments  24, 32
Proteolytic materials  32
Purpose of cleansing products & shampoos  109

## R

Remedies for hair damage  168
Relationship of hair type to hair properties  41
Relative humidity  32

## S

Saw palmetto  85
Scalp  61
    Moisture and TEWL  62
Sebaceous glands  65, 99
Seborrheic Dermatitis/Dandruff  76, 99
    Treatment of-  90
Senescent baldness  99
Shampoo damage mitigation  135

Shape of hair  48, 65
Shape of curly hair bulb  66
Shine  56
State of hair and scalp before treatment with conditioner  177
Static charge  55
Static electricity  55
Structure of hair schematic  9
Styling products  195
    Types  195
    Coconut oil water  196
    Curl enhancing smoothie  198
    Curling jelly  197
    JBCO water  196
    Setting lotions  199
    Smoothing gels  199
    Twist defining cream  197
Styling products for chemically straightened hair  205
    Anti-frizz leave-in conditioners  206
    Blow dry lotions  205
    Laminates  205
Surgical transplantation  91

# T

Telogen  54
Telogen effluvium (TE)  99
Tensile strength  32
    Wet hair  43
Tissue  99
Tissue types  99
Trace elements  32
Traction alopecia (TA)  100
Transepidermal water loss (TEWL)  100
Trichogram  100
Types of hair  38-40
Twists in hair  43

Type 1   38
Type 2   39
Type 3   40
Type 4   40
Types of conditioners   182
Types of detergents   116
Types of shampoos   141
Tyrosine   32

## V

Vertex   69, 72, 101
Vitamin A   89
Vitamin D   89
Vitamin E   89

## Z

Zinc   88

# NOTES

# NOTES

# NOTES

# NOTES

# NOTES

# NOTES

# NOTES

# NOTES